MAKING
Angels

A Story of Blessings on Our Journey
to Have Children after the Heartache of Infertility,
Miscarriage, and Late-term Pregnancy Loss

STACEY URRUTIA

Scripture quotations marked (NIV) are taken from the Holy Bible, New International Version®, NIV®. Copyright © 1973, 1978, 1984, 2011 by Biblica, Inc.™ Used by permission of Zondervan. All rights reserved worldwide. www.zondervan.com The "NIV" and "New International Version" are trademarks registered in the United States Patent and Trademark Office by Biblica, Inc.™

Paperback ISBN   978-0-9966871-0-2
eBook ISBN   978-0-9966871-1-9

Cover design by Sherwin Soy.
Cover photograph of boys courtesy of Stacey Urrutia.
Cover photograph of author courtesy of Brandy Angel Photography.

Printed in the United States of America

For more information about this book or to contact the author, please visit www.makingangels.com

"This book is written straight from the heart. It truly captures all the ups and downs that some couples unfortunately experience as they try to achieve their dreams of having a child. It is a must-read for couples who have experienced both difficulty and loss while trying to achieve this dream."
—Andrew A. Toledo, MD

To TCU and ASU, my earth angels:
May you always know how very loved you are.
It took me a while to learn that God is never late.
His divine plan unfolds in His perfect timing. I learned a lesson
in patience while waiting for our family to be complete.

To my beloved husband, Kevin, who inspired me to share our
story despite how painful it was at times.
Thank you for encouraging me to leave this legacy for our cherubs.
Through this journey we made together, you became not just a
partner to me, but a part of me.

And to my sweet Tess and our other angels.
I look forward to our heavenly reunion when the time is right.

CONTENTS

INTRODUCTION

I am writing this introduction as both a physician and as a patient. You see, I am a fertility specialist who works with couples like Stacey and her husband, Kevin. But my wife and I are also patients who went through many of the same trials and travails that you will read about in this book.

As I read *Making Angels*, what struck me most was the honesty with which Stacey describes her experience in her attempt to have children. This book starts with a brief description of Stacey's and Kevin's own journey, and their desire to help other couples who have found themselves walking this same path. What follows is a very accurate account of the Urrutias' progression from an innocent, naive couple excited to start their family to a couple beaten and battered by this difficult road which, ultimately, was successful for them.

Reading about Stacey's experiences evoked in me many different feelings. These emotions of sadness, anger, frustration and, finally, joy were brought about because of my own experience as both a physician *and* as a patient.

Stacey's memoir once again demonstrates that the journey itself is the most important lesson to be learned in a couple's quest for family. As Stacey points out in her book, sometimes couples can get lost in the process but, ultimately, faith and perseverance will prevail.

There are moments that you will read about in Stacey's

story that are oftentimes funny, but sometimes very gut-wrenching. Many of these moments brought tears to my eyes because they were so authentic. It is a very down-to-earth, straight-from-the-heart story that makes this book, in my opinion, mandatory reading for couples who find themselves on the emotional rollercoaster ride of infertility and recurrent pregnancy loss.

So, as you read this book, remember that while every couple's path to parenthood is unique, all can draw strength from the experiences this extraordinary woman shares in *Making Angels*.

Andrew A. Toledo, MD
CEO, Reproductive Biology Associates, and
    Husband of an Infertility Couple
Atlanta, Georgia

FOREWORD

This is a story about our journey to have a family. It was something that for a young healthy couple seemed like an obvious and simple path, and yet it turned out to be the most complex and trying time of our lives. Mostly young and naive, we had no idea how perilous and exhausting this journey would be. It's a quest that I wouldn't have wished on my worst enemy, and yet it's one that I would undertake again a hundred times over to have my boys.

Without my wife Stacey's determination and desire to have a family, it's likely that I would have never understood the magnitude of love one can feel for a child. That love has been the single greatest blessing of my entire life. It is something so unbelievable that I couldn't have imagined it in my wildest dreams. It's a devotion that words can't explain, and I believe you can't fully comprehend, until you are graced with a child.

Thank you, Stacey, for both giving me and being the love(s) of my life!

To our two earth angels, Tyler and Drew, thank you for the constant joy you bring us. Mommy and Daddy love you with all our hearts!

For the angels who have left us and gone on to a better place, you will always live in our hearts. It is in your honor that we will cherish all of life's blessings.

—*Kevin Urrutia*

PREFACE

YOU ARE NOT ALONE

This journey of ours—to create a family—is clearly special to *us*, because it is ours. But I am sharing it for two reasons: First, so that our children may one day read this and know exactly what we went through in an effort to bring them into this world. Second, and equally as important, to make this story available to those of you who have experienced similar difficulties and wrestle to understand them or relate to others as a result. The things people say, including close family and friends, may be well-intentioned. But as a woman who has been wounded by infertility and pregnancy loss, I feel that the comments have a sting to them that only others who have fought a comparable battle can empathize with.

The sufferings my husband and I endured give us the experience to help others with a similar fate. It is only because I have struggled through the same thing that I am qualified to offer you comfort in a way that is relatable. And for all of us who face these struggles, I believe we learn to persevere through them—to understand them, and eventually to embrace them. For out of the pain I have gained additional immeasurable gifts. Out of our tragedy arose a stronger relationship with God, the birth of our sons, and the drive to comfort others in the wake of their losses.

Our infertility and baby loss story has a happy ending...

but not without plenty of casualties and grief along the way. Many of you can sympathize with this—if you are trying to conceive but can't, or have had a miscarriage, or lost a baby shortly after birth, or have a daughter, sister, aunt, or friend who you know has lived through some version of this struggle to have children. My prayer is that by my sharing our story, you and your loved ones will know you too can survive despite this pain. Our journey has also been one of learning that there is a higher power in control of our lives. We might not always understand the function, influence, and omniscience behind that power, and that's okay. It doesn't mean I'm suggesting that you sit back and do nothing. I was the extreme opposite of that—the more things went wrong in our attempts to have children, the more I tried to control.

As a result I have indeed come full circle, to appreciate our journey rather than look back upon it with regret. It took me a long time to get there, even after we finally had children to call our own. When the loss of our five pregnancies was fresh, it seemed no one could relate to what I was feeling. I became inducted into a secret society of losers, an official member of the Those of Us Who Can't Bear Children Club. Women have been somewhat trained in our culture to quietly walk through life losing our babies (or trying to conceive them) and keep the disappointment to ourselves. That's a lot of pressure to put on a family. Other losses we bear are recognized publicly, so why not this one? The acknowledgment of a loss, whether it be death or even the loss of hope, is part of what defines its significance.

Please know that for any of you out there suffering

through infertility and pregnancy loss, or who have a family member or friend on a similar journey, we are crying with you or cheering for you. Whatever the outcome, you are not alone. Hindsight has allowed us to realize that we endured the adversity that came to us for the purpose of being able to console others. While I cannot change your circumstances, our story has equipped me with tools that may help lift your spirit and reassure you that there is a bigger meaning behind our similar sufferings.

With regard to calling my loved ones and lost babies "angels," I am fully aware from a biblical standpoint that I am not literally making angels. I am using the humanized sentimental version of that term. Each of us who has to endure the agony of losing a child grieves in our own way. We must find some sense of peace amid the pain. For my husband and me, referring to our children as angels came naturally. I do think they have a life unending, like that of an angel. But beyond that, they are infinitely pure and precious to us as we remember those babies who have passed and the ones who remain here on earth with us today.

So this is our story. I hope it inspires and encourages you to know you have found someone who has traveled a treacherous road to make a family and not only survived, but thrived. I hope the telling of our events provides insight and fosters understanding into the very real and sometimes raw feelings that accompany such a journey. Whether you too or someone you know has been on a similar path, I hope our story helps you fully appreciate the angels in your life.

ONE

OUR FIRST ANGEL

On February 21, 2001, I went to my rescheduled ob-gyn appointment. I missed the original appointment only days earlier because I was terribly ill. In fact, I had spent the past ten days in that condition. Surrendering to my failing health, I sequestered my wilting body to the living room couch for most of the episode. It was one of those rare occasions in my otherwise healthy and extremely active life that I can remember being so sick. The virus meandering its way through me had not been kind. Hacking and coughing until I nearly threw up, I had been running a high fever for days. My muscles were aching all over…this bug was more of a nuisance than just your typical winter virus.

My husband, Kevin, and I had recently moved from New York City to Alpharetta, Georgia. Seventeen weeks along in my first pregnancy, I had been to my new ob-gyn once for a brief visit to confirm my pregnancy, and another time for an interim checkup to confirm a heartbeat and look for regular embryonic development. Only a day shy of my thirtieth birthday, I was thrilled to be pregnant with our first child, as was Kevin. I had a list of both boy and girl names already constructed. The nausea that dominated my life for the past three months had finally faded away, and I was proudly displaying my rounded belly with a wardrobe of recently purchased maternity wear. For Dr. Michael Cohen's busy ob-gyn office, I was just another patient breezing through without much notice.

I was in the final interviewing process for a job with a local health-care marketing communications company. Having worked in the field of oncology for a decade, I felt my skills were well suited for the business. My background included preclinical research, pharmaceutical sales, and a stint in the popular dot-com industry, where I held a business develop-ment position for a start-up focused on oncology. If I secured this new position, I would be in charge of sales and business development. My medical knowledge combined with a sales background was a good fit.

At that point in our lives, Kevin and I were fully absorbed in our careers. We were constantly on the road for business and, sadly, we used our pagers as a means of sending messages about what city we were in or when we would be back home. My life was simpler at the moment, since I was between jobs, but Kevin, who was a medical device sales representative at the time, spent most of his days on the road covering all of Georgia, Alabama, and eastern Tennessee.

About a week earlier, I had called to tell my doctor's office that I was remarkably sick and asked to reschedule, since they probably didn't want my germs contaminating their waiting room. I asked some basic but concerned questions regarding the baby's health, wondering whether he/she could tolerate the virus coursing through me, given the horrible state I was in. The office staff reassured me that I was past the first trimester, and that babies can withstand mommies getting sick. They advised me to stay hydrated and get lots of rest. I felt fine with the advice at the time. Quite honestly, I think there are very few options for a pregnant woman fighting a virus. There likely wasn't anything else they could have said to me.

Days later, when I was still not recovering, my concern was mounting, so I called the ob-gyn office over the weekend and spoke to the doctor on call. I was even sicker and felt like I was going to die. I gave him a brief history. Again I was given the same advice.

I finally rebounded two days later, and the moment I felt good enough to get out, I called my doctor's office to ask to come in for my missed checkup. I was far enough along that I was hoping they would go ahead and do an ultrasound on this visit. They would check the health of the baby and just maybe, if I was lucky, I would get a sneak peek and find out the sex of the baby. I was apprehensive about how the baby was doing, since I had been so unwell; despite my concerns, I felt excited heading to the appointment. Our growing embryo should now look more like a baby than a tadpole. From my research, I knew the baby's cartilage was turning to bone, and his/her size was similar to a medium-size onion. I was disappointed Kevin couldn't join me, but as usual, he was on the road for work.

When I was finally called into the patient room, Dr. Cohen's nurse, Stephanie, greeted me warmly and began asking me questions and checking my vitals. I told her about how ill I had been as she listened for the baby's heartbeat as a matter of routine. She moved the fetal Doppler across my belly over and over again. I waited for the thundering sound to fill the room. The last time I had heard it I was reminded of galloping horses—*thud-thud, clip-clop, thud-thud, clip-clop*. After quite some time when she couldn't seem to find it, she casually asked me to go into the ultrasound room so she could see the baby's anatomy while she found the heartbeat.

"That baby is hiding in there! Let's go take a look," was her passing comment.

"Sounds good to me." I hopped off the exam table with enthusiasm and we relocated to the ultrasound room. Moments later I was stretched out on the table, getting the ultrasound I had hoped for. I saw one flash of our baby on the monitor; then Stephanie turned the screen away from me and told me she'd be right back while she went to get Dr. Cohen.

I always felt cold at the ob-gyn office. As the goose bumps emerged, I grew impatient just thinking about how long it might take to resume our ultrasound. I focused on seeing our developing baby and hearing his/her heartbeat. I couldn't wait to get a new photo and share it with Kevin the moment he came home. To my surprise, Stephanie returned with my doctor in less than a minute.

Dr. Cohen was a gracious and gentle man. He was

pleasant, with a happy demeanor that was almost contagious. As his patient, I could tell instantly that he loved what he did for a living. This day he was unusually quiet as he walked into the room, keeping our normal chitchat to an absolute minimum.

He quickly continued the ultrasound, staring intensely at the screen. As he moved the handheld device across my belly, he asked me a few questions, including whether I had felt the baby move at all. I told him I thought I had felt fluttering. I didn't know what type of movement was normal. I reminded him it was only my first pregnancy. Why was he asking me all these questions? Something about his attitude made me wonder whether everything was okay. Did the baby have a heart problem? Was he worried the baby had Down syndrome? My mouth turned so dry it was hard to swallow.

Dr. Cohen grabbed my hand and looked intently into my eyes. His face was dead serious as he leaned in to speak to me while I remained lying on the examination table.

"Your baby doesn't have a heartbeat. I'm so sorry." And finally, after some hesitation he uttered the words I feared hearing most: "You've lost the baby."

His words hung in the air, stuck there for me to absorb. It took a few seconds for me to process what I had just been told. Then a different kind of chill resonated through me. Breathless, I lifted my head off the pillow and propped up onto my elbows. I stared at him for a moment, as if magically his words could be reversed. I quickly shook my head back and forth, clearing the cobwebs that seemed to be cluttering my brain. Then the full impact hit me.

My heart pounded out of my chest, throbbing, beating

wildly, which made my baby's soundless heart even more silent.

Weeping softly, I told him how sick I had been. I informed him of all the phone calls I made to his office over the past week and a half. I desperately tried talking myself out of the nightmare. I mumbled nonsense about the series of events that had occurred in the past ten days, as if retelling it would turn back time and the doctors could do something, anything, to make our baby better. Surely I had heard him wrong. Surely this wasn't happening to me. This was the sort of thing that happened to other people. But nothing I said changed the outcome. I was still carrying our dead baby. My unblemished world began to collapse around me, tarnished with the loss of a child whose life I could no longer protect. I wiped the moisture from my face. My exterior shell appeared calm, but on the inside I was frantic to find a solution. I had always been able to fix things. My heart swelled with an aching I couldn't describe, bruised and beaten to a pulp. I was left numb.

I glanced over at the monitor, a viewing window into my child's world. The picture was no longer there. My mind returned to the last image I knew of our child. I visualized our baby on the ultrasound screen and remembered with such precision the way it was lying flat rather than curled up in the classic fetal position. I could see its perfectly formed body just resting there completely still. And I was the casket. Already guilt consumed me. As the lifeline for our baby, I had failed to perform the most fundamental task a mother can do.

I spent the next few minutes desperately trying to reach

Kevin on his cell phone. I knew he was in a surgical case, which meant he was unavailable while in the operating room. The medical device he sold was the first of its kind in the United States, and the FDA training guidelines for this particular device required that a company representative be present until the physician had completed the certification process. As such, Kevin was an important part of the team that helped surgeons perform lifesaving procedures. This made him unavailable for hours at a time. I sent a message to his pager along the lines of "BABY 911," followed by instructions to call me immediately on my cell or at Dr. Cohen's office. Because I couldn't reach Kevin, I called my parents. If I shared the loss with someone else, maybe it would dilute my pain.

I reached my father first and began crying harder. Between gasps, I finally got the words out.

"I can't believe it, but I lost the baby. We don't know why yet, but they did an ultrasound and there was no heart-beat."

"I'll stop what I'm doing here. Let me get Mom and we'll come in right away."

I am very close to my parents, and luckily they lived only an hour and forty-five minutes away, so they both dropped everything and headed toward my home. Eventually Kevin contacted me on a landline at the doctor's office. My body trembled as I shared the devastating news. Although he was distraught, his reaction was tempered, as it was his nature to be composed. In this crisis, Kevin's calmness provided a healthy dose of sanity for me.

It's strange, but I can't remember how I got home. I

probably waited for Kevin to pick me up so I wouldn't have to drive. This I know—it felt like an eternity between the time I learned of our baby's demise and the time our baby was removed from my womb. I remained in shock as I waited.

Before I left the doctor's office, Dr. Cohen inserted a special tubular piece of dried seaweed into my cervix. Evidently the seaweed absorbs water from the surrounding tissues and dilates the cervical canal. This process would help prepare my body for the scheduled D&E (dilation and evacuation) the following day.

That evening I felt unbearable heartache as constant waves of crying and disbelief washed over me. Although my family tried to comfort me, I preferred to be alone in my misery. Sharing the news with everyone hadn't made it better. Ironically, the more they tried to comfort me, the more self-blaming I became. Retreating to my bedroom, I buried myself deep under the covers, wishing at times my cocoon were my crypt. The responsibility of caring for this baby fell on me in full force. The safest shelter for our child should have been in my womb. Dr. Cohen's words gnawed at me like a mosquito that wouldn't stop its annoying high-pitched ringing in my ear…. "You've lost the baby. You've lost the baby."

I wrestled my way through the night, stroking my belly, telling our baby how sorry I was for not doing a better job or being a better mother. I don't know whether the overwhelming nausea I experienced was a side effect of my agony or my leftover pregnancy hormones.

I asked God a million times over, *Why? I want this baby so badly. Why choose me to lose a baby?* I had endless questions.

Did the baby suffer or feel any pain? Did he or she die slowly? Was there anything I could have done differently? How long had the baby been dead? Did I travel too much at work? Was I under too much stress? Did I lift something too heavy? How could a benevolent God leave me feeling so much pain? Was God even a loving God? As a child I was raised in a church environment where I had been taught to respect God out of fear rather than as a result of his unending love for me. Was this my punishment for things I had done wrong in my life? Did I deserve this?

The next morning was February 22, my thirtieth birthday.

My mood shifted from crushing grief to anger. The lack of answers infuriated me. I snapped at my family as they tried to console me once again. Nothing they could say or do was going to bring the baby back. We sat in the kitchen that morning, still trying to process what had happened. Multiple times my husband or parents tried to wrap their arms around me, but I pushed them away.

Before we left for the hospital, I quickly threw on some sweats and headed to brush my teeth. Our bathroom had double sinks. Kevin stood leaning over his, one hand bracing him on each side, his eyes shut and his head hung low. I began to brush. Vigorously. Furiously. Foaming at the mouth like a rabid animal, I looked at Kevin and uttered, "Happy fuckin' thirtieth." I am a properly raised, well-mannered lady in most circumstances, but at a time like this, it felt good to drop the F-bomb. My sarcasm startled him from his stance and he simply replied, "I'm so sorry."

At about six a.m., Kevin drove me to the hospital. The silence in the car was deafening. Upon checking in, I was bewildered that the hospital staff didn't pick up on the fact that I was about to lose a baby on my birthday. I realize that sounds completely self-centered, but it can't be every day that a woman walks into the hospital to lose her first baby on her thirtieth birthday. I'm sure everyone was just "being professional," or more likely they truly didn't notice.

As part of the prep for the D&E they gave me Versed (midazolam). It helps you forget the events surrounding the surgery. Apparently, Kevin tells me, after the Versed was well into my system I started singing nursery rhymes. The poor hospital staff had to suffer through that misery. I can't sing to save my life. To make matters worse, one of the songs was:

Oh, I wish I were a little bar of soap (bar of soap).
Oh, I wish I were a little bar of soap (bar of soap).
I'd a slippery and a slidey over everybody's hiney.
Oh, I wish I were a little bar of soap (bar of soap).

Seriously? Of all the things to sing? That was the one I picked? When I was a young child, this was a tune my brother and I would sing as a joke to be silly during bathtime. Allegedly the staff got a real kick out of it. I have no remembrance of it at all, thank goodness. On top of everything else I was feeling, I would have been totally embarrassed.

When I woke up from the procedure and was still in the recovery area, I felt tears streaming down my face. Funny how you can awaken from anesthesia and still your body is so emotionally tuned in that it knows what has happened before there is time to process it. I was crying before I was conscious of it. One of the nurses walked over to me and clasped my hand between hers.

"I'm sorry, sweetie," she murmured, pain in her voice.

There. It was said. Someone involved in the expulsion of our baby from my body finally acknowledged the loss I was experiencing. Besides Dr. Cohen, everyone else had been so robotic. They seemed so uncaring and callous, at least with specific regard to our miscarriage. Of course, they were just doing their jobs, and it was likely they saw this sort of loss more often than I realized. How should I expect sympathy from people who knew relatively little about me or my situation? Why should I expect them to give condolences to us? The staff had been kind in every other way.

She dabbed my face with a tissue.

"I'm sorry. I'm a little bit of a mess," I whispered. "I didn't want to lose the baby," I added. For some reason I felt the need to share with her that I had not had the D&E by choice.

For years after that, I wore mostly black on my birthdays, and muttered unkind words to myself as my parents, husband, family, or friends lovingly wished me a happy birthday. "Thank you." I would smile, but inside it made me squirm. I managed somehow to maintain a facade that everything was okay, but I felt disgusted in reality. It was death day to me. The day I lost our first angel.

When I think back to that dreadful day, one of the few regrets of my life is that I didn't spend a few more minutes looking at that ultrasound in Dr. Cohen's office. As it turns out, the lab that evaluated our loss surmised that the baby died from viremia. In other words, I was so sick that the baby died from the virus I had. Exactly what I was worried about. Dr. Cohen believed the baby probably died several days before I came to his office for the checkup, because they were unable to grow any cells in culture to better evaluate the cause of the loss. This also means that they could not tell us the gender of the baby. In a peculiar sort of way, that made it harder for me to put closure on things. I didn't have the ability to give our baby a name, and I longed for a better identity for him or her. The baby and I had spent the past eighteen weeks together. I had enough unanswered questions revolving around the circumstances of his/her death. It just seemed like the final blow to not even figure out whether I had lost a son or a daughter. In addition, due to the nature of a D&E, there were no remains for cremation or burial. Both my womb and my heart were hollow.

I spent much of my time feeling responsible for our loss. After all, it was my body that failed to protect our little one. Even worse, I tortured myself with constant thoughts of, What pain had the baby endured? How long had he or she suffered?

Intellectually, I knew it was not fair to put those pressures on myself. But with my emotions hitting me in the midst of it all, who else could I blame? Only me. For years my mother had told me what an easy time she had getting pregnant and carrying both my brother and me. Shouldn't it be that easy for me too?

To top things off, I dealt for months and months with the documents from our health insurance company. All the paperwork was labeled, "Abortion." I finally said something to one of the customer service reps as politely as I could.

"Perhaps you could consider creating a different code and term for pregnancy loss when it is an unintentional loss," I pleaded.

I calmly explained that the use of that term seemed cruel to me, because it insinuated that I chose to terminate the pregnancy. As if it were not difficult enough, there was the extra sting to my already self-inflicted indictment every time I saw the word on the paperwork.

"Well," he began in a calm voice, "this is the term the medical community uses, and how the procedure is coded whether or not the loss was made by choice." There was no changing it.

I thought about all the other women who would follow in my footsteps and be forced to deal with the same issue. While the medical community differentiated the loss of a pregnancy as either "induced abortion" or "spontaneous abortion," as a patient recovering from an unwanted loss of pregnancy, any association with the word "abortion" felt offensive.

Another difficulty in late-term pregnancy loss is that everybody already knows you're expecting. Because I am small in stature (only five-two, a hundred pounds), my pregnancy was obvious, and I had been wearing maternity clothes for quite some time. As a result, everywhere I went, people would make innocent comments about my changed belly size, or lack thereof. And then I would have to share the bad news over and over again.

One example of this took place in a local department store. I went shoe shopping just before I lost the baby. I had a pleasant conversation with the salesperson regarding my due date and other things we ladies love to talk about when there is excitement in the air for the impending birth of a baby. Not long after our loss, my mother drove me back to the store to run a quick errand.

I bumped into the same salesperson and she naively said to me, "Open your coat and show off that beautiful belly of yours!" In every possible way she meant to be sweet, but I had to tell her I had lost the baby. At every turn I dealt with explaining it.

The culminating event that epitomized exactly how painful this pregnancy loss was in my life occurred about ten days after I came home from the hospital. Although Kevin spent some time at home to deal with the loss himself and to comfort me as much as possible, he was pulled back to work only a few days later; he couldn't just ignore the busy surgical schedule that demanded his attention. In his absence, he felt there was no more suitable caregiver than my mother while I continued to recuperate. She stayed with me for several days until I felt I was ready to face the world alone. Roughly two weeks into my recovery she planned to leave Alpharetta and head back to her home. On the morning of her departure, I got out of bed at about seven a.m. and within twenty minutes I was on the floor in complete agony. I had an unexplained gut-wrenching pain in my belly. I called out for my mother, who fortunately heard me and came rushing into my bedroom.

"Please…get me to the emergency room!" I could barely get the words out.

She didn't hesitate and instantly helped load me into the car. It was rush hour on Georgia 400, the main highway we traveled to take us to the hospital. My mother helped me call Dr. Cohen on the way. As I spoke to him, she drove on the shoulder to avoid the heavy traffic. The pain was excruciating, and it sent me into a panic. I started to breathe too heavily and quickly; my arms began tingling, going numb. Dr. Cohen basically yelled at me (and rightfully so) to slow my breathing. I needed to be jolted out of my horrified state of mind. We talked about my symptoms. He told us he would have the emergency room staff ready when I arrived at Northside Hospital.

The slower breathing finally helped me settle down, and I regained a sense of control. But the loss of the baby followed by this inexplicable pain made me worry that something had gone seriously wrong. My mind raced into all the unknowns. *Is part of the baby still in me and my uterus is contracting to push it out?* I didn't think I was having contractions. And worse, *Is there some other related issue that will prevent me from being able to carry another baby?*

When I arrived at the hospital they were indeed ready for me, and rushed me into a room for examination and evaluation. After lots of poking and prodding and multiple ultrasounds, the consensus was that they didn't really have an answer. The pain medication running through my IV line finally kicked in. I was deeply relieved that they didn't see any major problem in my abdomen or, more specifically, my uterus.

I was eventually released late that evening with what remained a mystery diagnosis to everyone. One theory was that I had kidney stones, but nothing was conclusive. Dr. Cohen assured me he had definitely removed all the fetal tissue during the D&E, and there were no obvious remnants of the baby showing on the ultrasound.

It was a miserable time for me, though I had no idea how much worse it would get. This was only the beginning of our painful journey.

TWO

IN THE BEGINNING

As far back as I can remember, I wanted to be a mother. I didn't even need the handsome prince or a house with a white picket fence. I just wanted the kids. I suspect this stems from having two outstanding parents of my own. As a child I adored them, and I still do as an adult. They were loving, supportive, engaging, fun, and exciting to be around. I would consider them some of the nation's strictest parents. Consequently, I realize today that the values and morals they instilled in me as a child shaped me and prepared me for a world that is becoming increasingly hard to navigate. They taught me to be generous, kind, and thoughtful to others, and to always try my best. I learned to appreciate the blessings I had. As our family regularly toured European countries during my youth, I sensed that I became more patriotic than most other children. My parents were both active members of our community; they worked hard to raise money for our church and for arts and education in our area. They each led lives that were shining examples of how one should give back to family and society. I, probably like many other little girls, wanted one day to be a mommy just like my mother was to me.

I had a charmed childhood. I grew up in Hilton Head Island, South Carolina. Our family moved there from Newburgh, New York, in the early seventies, when very few people were full-time residents on the island. With the area having a population of only about five thousand, everything from grocery and clothes shopping to medical care basically mandated a trip to a more urban area. There was only one traffic light on the island, and a two-lane road that stretched from end to end. We typically made road trips to nearby cities like Savannah, Beaufort, or Charleston; stopping at a fast-food joint along the way was considered a very special treat. My father spent most of his years in Hilton Head working in real estate sales or development, and my mother was a stay-at-home mom, but she often had as long a day as my father, because she volunteered for so many organizations in the community.

My brother and I attended the public school system from kindergarten through twelfth grade, and my parents were heavily involved in making the public schools on Hilton Head some of the best in the state of South Carolina throughout the seventies and eighties. When we first moved to Hilton Head, the public schools were roughly ninety percent black and ten percent white. One of the fairly unique aspects of my childhood there was that as a white girl, I was a minority in school. Many of my best friends were black (as they called themselves), as were many of the educators and school leaders. I had tremendous respect for those authority figures, and for all they taught me.

I was raised in a household with two loving parents, had two sets of grandparents nearby, and five great-grandparents in my life. I grew up able to spend time on the beach, and was an avid lover of nature, which was easy in a place like Hilton Head. My mother seemed to know everything about the plants and animals that surrounded us, and she spent hours telling us about the beautiful nature of our island. I was an athletic kid, and by the age of eight I was playing in United States Tennis Association (USTA) tournaments. My mother and father spent a generous amount of money on tennis lessons for my older brother and me. Hilton Head was a great place to foster a tennis career. My father would often wake us up early, and we would head to the neighborhood tennis court to get one hour of practice in before the start of the school day. My patient and dedicated mother would take us to tournaments all over South Carolina throughout the summer months, and eventually we were both good enough that we competed in the Southern regional tournaments as well as national competitions.

In the meantime at school I was having success as a straight-A student, becoming class president, helping my high school tennis team win the state championships, and competing in science fairs. As a junior in high school, I won the International Science and Engineering Fair, an award that allowed me to attend the Nobel Prize ceremonies in Stockholm, Sweden. That, combined with my tennis and academic achievements, put me on the cover of *USA Today* as one of their 1989 All-USA High School Academic (First Team) top-twenty students in the country.

I later attended Princeton University, a school that further shaped me. While I was at Princeton, my senior thesis as a premed biology major involved wound healing and neurosurgery on rats. I had always intended to go to medical school in order to become a neurosurgeon. But I made a conscious decision during college to change from premed to planning for a career in health care that did not include becoming a physician. I did this with the notion that it would increase my chances of being a great parent to my future children. Throughout my decision-making process, I had at least three very successful surgeons warn me that I would either be a great surgeon and a horrible mother, or a horrible surgeon and a decent mother, or very mediocre at both. Something would have to give. The message was loud and clear: The lifestyle of a (hopefully one day) accomplished neurosurgeon would not allow for great mothering—at the least I would be less attentive simply based on my work hours. I would not be around enough to be the parent I imagined. Couple that with the financial changes that were taking place in the health-care system at the time, such as the rising cost of medical malpractice insurance, and it influenced me in such a way that I felt discouraged from becoming a surgeon.

The other influence in my life with regard to a career was my father. While I was growing up, he had a job that allowed for flexibility in his schedule. He worked long, hard days, but often enough he could swing by to see me compete on the tennis court. I always appreciated his work-life balance and aspired to achieve the same for myself.

My course was forever altered, and I didn't even apply to medical school. My small-animal surgical skills did not go to waste, however; I carried them into my first job working for Hoffmann-La Roche, a Swiss global health-care company. I secured a position in their pharmaceutical division, working in the preclinical Research and Development Department of Oncology.

In hindsight, I have realized that there are many women today who live their lives with both a demanding career and an active role in mothering. More than once that has made me question my decision not to become a doctor. Nevertheless, after graduation, my career choice was cancer research. I found it was a way to combine my love for science with my surgical skills. My job gave me a sense of pride as a collaborator in the battle against cancer, and because of my work hours, it also provided for a quality of life that was amenable to my being a deeply engaged mother.

THREE

AN UNEXPECTED LOVE

My career in research was going well; however, I felt limited by not having a doctorate degree. Plus, for reasons associated with the health of the lab animals (I worked with rodents that were susceptible to infection), my job mandated that I work in a shower-in/shower-out barrier facility. On a daily basis, and sometimes more than once a day, I was required to shower and dress in laboratory clothing. Before entering the animal room I strapped a ventilation system around my waist. It connected by way of a hose to a biosafety helmet that I placed on my wet hair. After completing my work, I showered before re-dressing in civilian clothes. Two years of that became cumbersome, and for much of my day I felt cut off from the rest of the world. But the extra time and schooling for a Ph.D. didn't seem worth it to me, so I made a move from preclinical research and development to pharmaceutical sales. In the meantime, my love life took an interesting turn. I met a guy on a blind date and we quickly fell for each other. He was from New Jersey but went to law school in Oregon, so we had a relationship that was passionate but long-distance. In less than a year we were engaged. As we planned our lives together, we often talked about our future children and the names we liked for them. So I was taken by great surprise when one day my then-fiancé questioned me about having children. I was crystal-clear about what I wanted, and explained that even if I could not have them biologically, I would definitely have a surrogate or adopt. It was simple: My life's future would include children regardless of how I got there. My fiancé was apparently taken aback by this.

"You mean if I decided I didn't want children, then you would leave me?" he asked.

"Absolutely," I said without hesitation.

I explained that I had always wanted children, and I assumed he did too. He had never indicated that there would be a future for the two of us that didn't include them. I was his first serious relationship, and his fickle attitude toward such a momentous topic deeply concerned me. In the time we dated, and during nearly a year of our engagement, it was no secret that I wanted to be a mother. For me, this was a deal breaker. That night we ended our relationship. I have never looked back or second-guessed myself on that one. I'm sure it was a good decision for him, too. I knew marriage would have too many unpredictable twists and turns without our being in such opposition on this matter.

Even though I was only twenty-five, my biological clock

was ticking. Plus, I felt like "tainted goods." Who would want a girl who had failed at an engagement already? My mother and father were married at ages twenty-three and twenty-four, respectively, and my mother got pregnant with my brother on their honeymoon. She had my brother when she was twenty-four, and delivered me by the time she was twenty-seven. I was twenty-five years old and didn't even have a boyfriend.

The funny thing is, as people say, "Love finds you when you least expect it." The day after I broke off the engagement, I started a new job for the pharmaceutical giant Abbott Labs, in New York City. Plans for my first week on the job included a company-wide meeting at an airport hotel in Newark, New Jersey. By eight a.m. I was on one of the pay phones in the lobby asking my ex-fiancé to remove his things from my apartment and meet me later that week with his spare key. I was, not surprisingly, puffy faced from a long night of crying, and that last phone call didn't help the cause. I couldn't believe what was happening, though I knew it was the right decision.

After the call, I headed to a common room where all divisions from the company were gathering for breakfast. I sat down with two fellow employees whom I had met over the course of my training period. Little did I know that Kevin was there and spotted me from afar, and, God bless him, despite my red, swollen, tearstained face, he says he knew right away he wanted to meet me. He now tells the story that when he saw my face he figured I had either been crying or had the worst allergy attack he had ever seen. Nevertheless, later he asked the women I was sitting with (who were friends of his) about me.

One of them spoke up and told him, "We can introduce you to her, but she has some baggage. She just broke off an engagement. You don't really want to meet her, do you?"

"Well, how recently did they break up?" he wondered.

"Last night!" they blurted out almost in unison.

Despite that news update, Kevin suggested they bring me to an upcoming social outing he and a few friends had in mind. They wanted a group to meet on a ship that toured the waters surrounding Manhattan.

One girl added, "We're not so sure we want to bring her. She's not much fun to be around right now."

Kevin gave his rebuttal: "Cut the girl some slack. She broke off an engagement less than twenty-four hours ago. What do you expect?"

Luckily, Kevin had just ended a five-year relationship himself, and he had a good understanding of what I was feeling at that very moment. A couple weeks later a group of our mutual business colleagues planned to gather on the booze cruise. Kevin convinced the girls to invite me along. Initially I was reluctant to go. I was stuck in my own pity party, wounded from my broken engagement. But with some prodding, I decided it would be emotionally healthy to get out socially, even if I pretended to have a good time. Kevin and I met shortly after arriving on the boat. We talked for hours that night. I told him right away about my broken engagement, and he told me about his recently failed long-term relationship.

I explained that I felt almost asexual—completely uninterested in anyone. For whatever reason, that did not turn him off, and we laughed for hours, exchanging jokes and stories and having a great time. I forgot how sad I had been. And since I really didn't care about how I looked or what he or anyone else thought of me that night, I was as authentic as could be. I didn't have any of the concerns a single girl would normally have when talking to a handsome man. Kevin and I traded contact information and made loose plans to be in touch. As I walked home that night my cheeks ached from the smile that hadn't left my face all evening.

For the next several weeks and months we talked on the phone quite a bit. That was rare for me; I was not big into long phone conversations with men. But whenever Kevin called, it seemed we had so much to discuss and share. Our dialogue was casual and easy, as if I had known him for years already. Although Kevin also lived in New York City, his apartment was far enough away that simply bumping into each other was not going to happen. Those phone calls were a good way for us to get acquainted without the pressure of dating.

Two months later, he finally asked me to come to a party at his apartment that he and his roommate were hosting. I was extremely hesitant until my two girlfriends from work said they planned to go. I had become better friends with them at this point, and I considered them my safety net. Little did I know that Kevin was working his magic behind the scenes, as he was the one persuading the girls to bring me along.

To this day, I remember climbing the steps to his apartment, staring up at him as he greeted me with a big smile. *What was I thinking? This guy is really cute! How did I not notice this before?* Standing before me was a handsome man. He was about five-ten, with an athletic build. Despite his casual dress, he had a bit of a *GQ* look. His hair was styled straight back, and I noticed his slightly olive complexion. Over the past several months we had spoken so many times, but never in person, so I had essentially forgotten his good looks. In that moment I realized I was finally no longer so brokenhearted. I could see past the heartache and get back into life again. It felt good to be interested in dating someone. Later that night, Kevin played the guitar and sang to me. He was trying to woo me with his talents, and it was working.

In the months following that night, I learned more about Kevin's family. Born to Cuban immigrants, he was a first-generation American. His mother came to the United States when she was fourteen, and his dad was nineteen when he made the journey over. They both fled from Cuba to escape Castro's rule. Initially hoping to go back to Cuba someday, they realized life there was changing in a way that made them not want to return. Not too long after my father-in-law, Raul, arrived in the States, he met Maria, my mother-in-law. They had a traditional Cuban courtship—chaperoned dates until they were married, when Raul was twenty-four and Maria was twenty. Several years later they were blessed with a baby boy, and only thirteen months after that they were fortunate to have a little girl. They raised their family in an apartment in Forest Hills, New York.

Not only did Kevin's parents leave Cuba, but a good number of his relatives made their way to the States too. Kevin was surrounded by both sets of grandparents, multiple aunts and uncles, and cousins. Much like my family, they enjoyed big family gatherings around meals, and had a strong focus on education in their household. In Cuba, between both families, they had owned a private school, several pharmacies, ocean-front property, and an apartment building. They were forced to give everything up, and worked hard to begin their new lives in another country.

Kevin, a native New Yorker, grew up speaking Spanish in his home. At age three he learned English in bits and pieces by playing with other toddlers in their apartment building. He perfected the language once he went to school. He was enrolled at a public school for kindergarten, and attended a private Catholic grammar school for grades one through eight. The following year he was accepted to Archbishop Molloy High School (then an all-boys school), where he completed his secondary education. After graduation he went to college at St. John's University, where he received a degree in marketing.

Kevin's childhood was radically different from mine in that I was raised in the quiet and peaceful beach town of Hilton Head Island, while his youth was spent navigating the streets and uncertainties that came with living in crime-ridden 1980s-era New York City. Kevin told me true stories from his adolescence that in my childhood existed only in movies. While I struggled to relate to his upbringing, I admired him—and his parents for raising the successful young man he has become. The obstacles he overcame were not insignificant.

One thing I started to understand early in our courtship was what I called "Cuban time." My first exposure to this was when Kevin and I arrived at his parents' house for what I thought was a noon get-together. When we strolled through the door at twelve fifteen p.m., I was concerned about being late. On the car ride to his parents' home, Kevin had insisted it wasn't a big deal that we were running behind. At nearly two p.m., the other guests still had not made an appearance. I questioned Kevin as to why they were so late, and wondered whether his parents were upset or offended by the delay in their arrival. He explained that it was typical in the Cuban culture to operate this way. That was brand-new to me, and took a little getting used to.

After a year of dating, and nearly a year of engagement, we tied the knot. When I least expected it, love had arrived. At the rehearsal dinner on our wedding weekend, I made a toast to "my Dennis," as our friends jokingly called Kevin. He was, after all, my rebounder, like Dennis Rodman, the seven-time NBA leading rebounder.

We half jokingly contemplated sending out a separate set of wedding invitations to Kevin's side of the family, with the start time of the wedding listed an hour earlier than the actual time. I knew my parents would think it was no joke if people breezed into the church during the ceremony. My sweet mother-in-law must have said the right thing to all the Cubans, though, because when Kevin arrived one hour early at the church, his entire family was already seated in the pews. We've had a good laugh about that many times over, but I was grateful for her persuasion that day. Over the years I have really grown to love Kevin's family. I have great respect for them, and I admire their passion and spirit. They are solid, good people whom I am lucky to call my family.

Kevin is the start of my story. The real beginning of how I see my life now. I thank God for him every day, and for the patience he has had with me on our voyage together. We never anticipated the ups and downs our life in partnership would have, but I feel truly blessed to be sharing it with him.

Not long after we were married, a friend of mine joked with me about the difficulty in how to pronounce his last name, Urrutia. Admittedly, it was tough. In fact, in our early months of dating I would sometimes call his work voice mail just to hear his recorded name so I could practice saying it correctly.

"You must love him an awful lot to take that last name," my friend kidded.

"Yes, I do. I do love him that much." I smiled.

On our fifteen-year anniversary, I told Kevin, as I always do, how dearly I love him. But this time it was different, because I wanted him to understand more than ever that during our time together I have come to love him as a part of me, not just a partner to me. It is that entwinement, that sense of being truly one, that has allowed us to triumph over the challenges we've faced together.

FOUR

TIME TO START A FAMILY

Life during our first few years of marriage was a blur. Although we were living in New York City, our wedding in August of 1998 took place in the little town of Greensboro, Georgia. Our friends thought we were totally crazy, since the only Greensboro even most Georgians know of is in North Carolina. However, my parents had moved to Greensboro in 1995, so we began visiting them while we were dating. It is a lovely small-town community centered around golf and picturesque Lake Oconee. To say the least, it is remote, and although it is much more developed now (it actually has a grocery store, a movie theater, and a Ritz-Carlton Lodge), at the time we loved how serene and charming it was. We felt it was the perfect retreat for a weekend wedding.

Everyone asks this question: What did you do with all your time before you had kids? Well, we worked. And then we worked some more. We both had jobs that kept us on the road constantly. Although we were employed by pharmaceutical companies when we first met, within a short period of time we both made career moves that basically left us seeing each other on weekends. Kevin went to work for a large medical-device company. I was at a dot-com start-up company in the health-care industry. We both had the desire to live in the South-eastern United States, where we felt the cost of living and quality of life would be better for us. Though my company was based in New York City, I had negotiated permission to live elsewhere. Only one year after we were married, Kevin was offered a job in the Atlanta area, giving us the chance to relocate. We moved to a fabulous family community in Alpharetta, Georgia.

While I had been eager to get pregnant for quite some time, Kevin was more hesitant. He knew adding children to our lives was a change that could not be undone. He very much wanted children, but wasn't in any rush to change our family dynamic. As a working couple with no children, we occasionally joined each other on weekend business trips; impromptu travel was a simple reality in our household, a luxury and freedom he appreciated. His attitude toward pregnancy was that we were a young, healthy couple who should easily be able to conceive. But there was great disparity between us on this subject. I pushed for getting pregnant sooner, knowing that sometimes it can take months before couples conceive. My twenty-nine-year-old body wasn't getting any younger. I always imagined our family having two children, and I knew the odds for having fewer complications for me and our babies were best if I could be finished having children by the time I was thirty-five. As I calculated my future, it meant we needed to get the process going. It took me nearly a year of persuading him before he conceded.

The first couple of months we tried getting pregnant we didn't make any special attempts to conceive. I wasn't taking my temperature or using ovulation predictor kits. Just ceasing our birth control was the effort we made. By the third month, I had a new game plan. After a visit to my local drugstore, I arrived home with several packs of ovulation-predictor kits. A thorough reading of the fine print allowed me to become acquainted with the instructions as well as gain a newfound knowledge of conception. Despite my biology background, the literature taught me about the various phases of my menstrual cycle, the details of which were much more important to me now than they had ever been in school.

Later that month, we were pregnant with our first baby. Relieved that our waiting time to conceive had been only three months, I secretly questioned whether I had overreacted in my eagerness to get pregnant. Regardless, I was grateful for our circumstances. Kevin shared in my excitement but admitted to being nervous about becoming a father.

I quickly welcomed the idea of having a child on the way. I began reading books about pregnancy but, after perusing a few of them, decided it was best to leave the literature on the shelf. There were so many things one could experience throughout a pregnancy, most of which only raised concerns I hadn't bothered to consider. I am enough of a worrier naturally that I didn't feel it was advisable to educate myself any further. Moving forward, if there was something in question, I either asked a friend who had already been pregnant or I called my doctor's office.

I was overjoyed by the mere idea of what my future family would look like, and it took every bit of self-control to keep our good news private for even a short time. Browsing through maternity magazines and checking out items at online baby stores was a routine exercise during my downtime. My enthusiasm was tempered by extreme nausea that I experienced throughout the day. There were several times at work where I wasn't sure I would make it through a presentation without vomiting. I got nervous just thinking about how to tell the client I might need to bolt out of the room for fear of throwing up in front of everyone. I couldn't disclose my pregnancy—I hadn't even told my family or my employer yet.

Luckily, the Thanksgiving holiday came only a few weeks after we conceived. Many of our relatives were gathered at my parents' house to enjoy the celebration together. My dad had built a roaring fire, and the smell of a perfectly roasted turkey filled the air. Just before we were about to say the blessing, Kevin and I summoned our family around the hearth and made our big announcement. We were pregnant! This child would not only be our first baby, but it would also be the first grandbaby for both sets of grandparents. My mother admitted she had been wondering when we would get around to making some grandchildren for everyone.

In the months that followed, I relished every detail of my pregnancy. Collections of ultrasound photos were pinned up around the house, baby names were being discussed, my growing belly forcing me into a new wardrobe. Kevin became comfortable with the idea of being a father. Whenever possible he would join me at the doctor's office. At night as we lay in bed he would stroke his hand over my ballooning belly and speak to the baby. It always began with, "How you doin'?" said facetiously in a strong New York accent. Our conversations were filled with dreams of our little one's future. I couldn't wait to see Kevin as a daddy.

At about sixteen weeks pregnant the nausea that consumed me finally faded away and I felt like a new woman. I had an appetite, energy, and was beginning to consider all the baby items we would need in only a few short months. My purchasing was limited by one thing—we didn't yet know if the baby was a boy or a girl. I decided to hold off on making any plans for the baby's room until after I learned the baby's sex. By week seventeen of my pregnancy, what started as a bad cold turned into a horrendous sickness—the awful virus that would have such devastating results. Only a week later, a day shy of my thirtieth birthday, our hearts were broken when we lost our first little angel. Dr. Cohen's words, "You've lost the baby," echoed in my head for months following our tragedy.

There was much to recover from. It was not only the physical recuperation from having the D&E, but also the conversations with everyone from close family members to practical strangers that made the loss of the baby so difficult.

The manner in which Kevin and I dealt with the loss

differed as well. While he was certainly devastated, his body had not experienced the hormonal fluctuations mine had. He didn't harbor the guilt that was an enormous emotional burden for me to bear. And because he didn't carry the baby, he had fewer conversations that required he explain our loss to others.

That being said, in Kevin's role as a salesperson, he was expected to be warm, engaging, and enthusiastic. He had happily shared the news of our pregnancy with many of his colleagues and customers. For weeks after we lost the baby he had to explain his somber mood.

The best remedy for my depressed state of mind was to focus on getting pregnant again. Kevin agreed that as long as it was physically safe for us to try, we should attempt to make another baby. We ran into a hurdle when I had a regular ob-gyn checkup. Given my late-stage pregnancy loss, Dr. Cohen wanted to check my reproductive health by performing both an ultrasound and a sonohysterogram; the latter was a procedure to look inside my uterus to check for scarring, masses like fibroids and polyps, or any abnormal shape or structure in my anatomy. During the exam, the uterus is filled with a saline solution. The saline expands the endometrial cavity and allows for a better assessment. Images are viewed by ultrasound to allow for evaluation.

While my ultrasound revealed nothing unusual, Dr. Cohen found a lesion in my endometrial cavity. Knowing that I was trying to get pregnant, he felt it was best that he remove the mass that could later become a problem if I conceived. I underwent a hysteroscopic procedure to remove the growth.

The procedure was uncomplicated, and fortunately all he found was a benign polyp.

Shortly after the surgery, I was relieved we were given permission to try to get pregnant again. Feeling pressure from the surgical delay, I did not waste a moment. I immediately purchased three packs of ovulation test kits and started peeing. I religiously arose from my bed every morning and checked the test stick. Since we got pregnant quickly and easily using those devices the first time around, I figured this would be a fairly uncomplicated process for us.

The first morning the ovulation test stick indicated I was about to ovulate, the clock read four a.m. It happened to be the morning Kevin and I were getting ready to fly from Georgia to Hawaii for an award trip he won at work.

Kevin walked into the bathroom, only one eye open, and nearly bumped into me.

"Turn around," I demanded. "The little blue line says this is our time to try making a baby, and we have to travel all day. You have five minutes to make it happen." Kevin reacted with a sarcastic chuckle but sauntered back to the bed. There's nothing like performing under pressure. Needless to say, we tried our best. Afterward I used Kevin's shower time to sit with my legs in the air, hips propped up at just the right angle, hoping that would boost my fertility. While there may not be any real medical evidence that this increases the odds of conception, it certainly can't hurt to improve your luck and give gravity a helping hand.

We arrived in Hawaii and Kevin felt our morning's events were funny enough to share with his colleagues, referring to our early morning interlude as the "Blue Stick Special." We all had a good laugh about it. I defended my position literally and figuratively. Sadly, we did not conceive that month or even the next five.

I became obsessed with the goal of getting pregnant. I used such a profuse number of ovulation-predictor tests, I should have bought stock in the companies that manufacture them. On days I performed home pregnancy tests, I found myself checking the used test stick in the trash can, hoping that somehow I hadn't read it correctly and that, if given enough time, the positive pregnancy line would eventually appear.

Kevin did not exactly appreciate the fervor with which I wanted to conceive again. He also grew frustrated by the lack of spontaneity in our sex life. While initially the idea of baby making had its appeal, for both of us it quickly grew more into a job than a joy. I was willing to do anything to adjust our schedule so we could be together and try to make a baby. He was more relaxed about it, and preferred to leave it up to nature alone as to when we would conceive. At one point I interacted with a female perinatologist (a physician who works within obstetrics, concerned with the care of the fetus during complicated or high-risk pregnancies) who informed me of the terms she had developed over time when referring to couples who have a hard time conceiving. "I call it 'sex without a cause' and 'work fucking.'" I was startled by her candor, but completely related to it. I think all couples, at first, have a romantic notion that making love to a husband or wife for the purpose of procreating will be the ultimate act of togetherness for the sake of family. But after enough failed attempts and scheduled sex around ovulation time, intimacy that was once pleasurable becomes associated with a task—to the point that it can feel like a chore in many ways.

Shortly after the loss of our first pregnancy, I started a new job. The New York-based Internet company I was working for had gone out of business, and I found employment at a health-care marketing communications firm in the Atlanta area. After going nearly a month without work, I was excited to have a busy and challenging career again. I was mentally healthier being employed. It gave me other goals, and was a welcome distraction from my focus on conception. The combination of our miscarriage and my being out of work had not been easy on our marriage. I had too much free time to become absorbed in the trauma of our loss. I suspect Kevin felt relieved that I was busy at work again.

My new boss and I often traveled together for business meetings. As we prepared to head out of town, I knew my window for pregnancy testing would overlap with our trip, so as every overeager woman would do, I brought along several home pregnancy tests. I had given my body more than four months' recovery time since the miscarriage and had just resumed exercising on a regular basis. I figured that getting physically fit would help my body scare away any nasty viruses in the upcoming winter. I joined my boss for a workout in the hotel gym. After a quick run on the treadmill (and lots of water for easy peeing), I headed back to my hotel room and went straight to the bathroom.

As I had done numerous times before, I sat on the toilet

and carefully watched as my urine saturated the test strip. I placed the test on the bathroom counter next to me and hovered on the seat while waiting for the urine to travel up the stick. My eyes fixated on the runway where the prognostic indicator lines were located.

I was pregnant for sure. The lines on the pee stick told me so! I felt awkwardly alone discovering I was finally pregnant, yet unable to share my news with anyone. Telling Kevin in person seemed much better than over the phone, so for the next couple days on the road I repeated the pregnancy test four more times just to make sure I was still pregnant. I would have happily peed on a test stick every time I went to the bathroom for the pure joy of seeing that magical pink pregnancy line appear. When I returned home, I went into the ob-gyn's office to confirm with a blood test, and as expected, all five test sticks were truthful. This time I was sure we were having a baby! It was after hearing back from the doctor's office that I finally told Kevin our good news. It may sound strange that I waited a few days to tell him, but after all we had been through in the past year, I wanted to be certain about the test results. The timing of hearing back from the ob-gyn coordinated well with Kevin's return from business travel.

He walked through the door and I already had one of his favorite dinners on the table. I handed him a glass of wine, we took our seats, and I raised my glass of milk high in the air. "You're going to be a daddy again!" I belted out over chicken cutlets, rice pilaf, and a green salad.

A wide smile took over his face, and he leaned across the table to kiss me. "Congratulations to us!" he cheered back with genuine enthusiasm. I related to him the series of events that had occurred over the course of the past few days, assuring him that because of the blood test, we could feel confident with the results. My tone was somewhat apologetic, as I confessed that I had been hiding the pregnancy from him until the ob-gyn's office confirmed it. He was understanding of my decision.

That evening we crawled into bed exhausted from our long workweek. Kevin pulled me up close to him so he could spoon me from behind. As he gently caressed my belly, we whispered to each other like teenagers in love. Were we having a boy or a girl? Would he/she like sports or music or art? Would our little one resemble Kevin or me? There were so many things to contemplate about our child's future. I barely slept that night as thoughts of our baby percolated through my mind.

FIVE

EARLY DOESN'T MEAN EASY

Once I confirmed my pregnancy, I was determined to be as healthy as possible and make sure I didn't get sick this time around. After sharing the good news with Kevin I called my dearest family and friends and let them in on our secret. I decided to wait until I was farther along in my pregnancy before letting everyone at work know.

I made a conscious effort to eat healthy while attempting to cater to my ongoing nausea. One day, only a week after being enamored with the news of our pregnancy, I left work around noon to indulge in an Asian chicken salad from a local restaurant. As I sat at the table, a strange sensation demanded my attention. There was moisture in my underwear. My heart skipped a beat. Abruptly I got up from the table and hurried to the nearest bathroom. Finding a stall, I paused for a moment and inhaled deeply, holding the oxygen in. I bowed my head and closed my eyes. *Breathe, Stacey. It might be okay. Just breathe.* I blew out the air, prepared for whatever I would discover. I wiggled my clothing down over my hips and stared at my panties. The curse of bright red streaks in my underwear was a reliable sign: This pregnancy was coming to an end, or had already expired. My soaring dreams for both the baby growing in me and the family I longed for came to a crashing halt yet again. I leaned forward against the stall and braced my head. I closed my eyes and wished away what I had just witnessed. I peeked down, only to find that the blood was still there as I fought to accept this new reality.

In defiance of what I had seen, only a few hours later I rushed home from work to take another pregnancy test. My heart pounded out of my chest as I anticipated the result. Confirming my fears, the pink "yes, you're pregnant!" line was getting weaker. Downstairs, I could hear Kevin arrive home from work. Up until then I'd held my emotions in, but seeing my husband and knowing what I needed to confess put me over the edge. Tears cascaded down my cheeks as I greeted him. Kevin cradled me in his arms while listening to what had happened. Our first pregnancy loss had occurred so late in gestation that we never predicted we would lose one this early, or even lose another pregnancy at all. Both of us crushed and grief-stricken, Kevin insisted that we make a few calls to substantiate our concerns. I phoned both my doctor and a friend's father, a well-respected ob-gyn. They each confirmed the painful truth: I was losing this baby too. I could expect a heavier than usual period as I went through the process.

In the days following our loss, I remained weepy. Kevin,

by contrast, was mostly filled with anger and frustration. While my devastation fueled me to work harder and faster at getting pregnant again, he became slightly disenchanted with the idea. He wasn't outright opposed to continuing our quest, but I think he saw how depressed I was, and desired to appease me by agreeing to whatever it was I wanted.

I remember that one of the hardest emotions to combat even then, after only two losses, was dealing with being around other pregnant women. It was one of the few times in my life that I had ever felt envy—true envy. I have always prided myself on feeling happy for others and not being jealous of what they have. Wanting to have a baby and watching others bear children while I failed was agonizing. All my life, if I put my mind to something and worked hard at it, I was able to achieve my goal.

Yet I couldn't carry out one of the seemingly most basic functions of the female body: reproduction. I couldn't successfully bring a baby into this world. There were teenage girls unwittingly getting pregnant in the backseats of cars. I'm pretty sure they weren't holding their legs up in the air for twenty minutes after sex, and yet they could conceive and carry a baby to term. Why couldn't I? I was a five-foot-two-inch, slim, healthy, active, and overall fit young woman. What was wrong with me? I was doing everything right and more, and it still wasn't working. To make matters worse, most of my colleagues at work were women of childbearing age. It seemed we always had someone pregnant roaming around the office. I sensed that those women were tuned in to my delicate state of mind, but it didn't change the circumstances. I yearned to be pregnant just like them, and only by the grace of God did my envy not prevent me from being truly pleased for them.

My despair was exaggerated by the attitudes of some of our friends. Some pregnant woman I interacted with would fuss about their growing bellies and the additional weight gain accompanying their pregnancy. Others who were further along would complain that they were tired of being pregnant, and wished they could deliver early. I would have happily given my right arm to get (and stay) pregnant, gain a few pounds, and give up a good night's sleep. One specific couple we spent a lot of time with already had two kids and had just found out they were pregnant with a third. They knew we were struggling to start a family. Their most recent pregnancy was an "oops" baby, and they made no secret of letting everybody know it. They whined and bemoaned repeatedly, openly admitting that they didn't want another child. At that time, they gathered together with our next-door neighbors and us for regularly scheduled Friday-evening "game nights." This was a guaranteed good time, except that this one thing was becoming increasingly difficult for me.

One particular evening after the couple's incessant lamenting about their newest pregnancy, I finally spoke up. "Well, some of us in the room are experiencing a truly hard time having a baby. If you really don't want your next child, I'll be more than happy to take it." My tone indicated that I meant what I said. I think that finally shut them up. Or at least that conversation stopped around me.

The other exchange that repeatedly took place in our lives was when neighbors asked, "Why did you buy such a big house when it's just the two of you?" We owned a five-bedroom home in a community that included an elementary school at the entrance. People who didn't know us very well couldn't figure out why we'd lived there for so long and yet had no children. We would comically answer, "We're DINKYs. You know…Double Income, No Kids Yet," which always seemed to break the ice and get a good laugh. It was easier than explaining one bedroom for us, one for a home office, one guest bedroom, and space for the two children we longed to have. And it was certainly simpler and less emotional than explaining our two failed pregnancies.

After my second loss, I was told we could try to conceive without waiting a few months, so we went right back to "work." My determination to conceive and carry a baby only continued to grow, and Kevin was a willing participant. He knew I had a mission, and while he wasn't as eager as I was to make things happen quickly, he also knew the sooner we could get pregnant and stay pregnant, the sooner this would no longer be an obstacle for us to overcome. I used the ovulation-predictor kits, and luckily my optimal days for making a baby fell at a time when both Kevin and I were in town. I checked and rechecked my calendar, anxiously counting down the days leading up to my home pregnancy test date. I planned, as a matter of routine by now, to test six days before I was to have a missed period. I had learned the test kits were capable of indicating a pregnancy quite early in my cycle.

That morning I was awakened by my eagerness to figure out whether we were pregnant. I crawled out of bed, careful not to wake Kevin or our dog, Jewel. Grabbing the box that

STACEY URRUTIA

contained pregnancy test sticks, I quietly unwrapped one. I knew the concentrated hormones in my morning urine would have the best chance of telling me whether I was pregnant or not. I held my breath as I watched the urine creeping up the stick.

A line indicating pregnancy hormone was barely visible, but I could see it nonetheless. It was positive! Sitting on my toilet, alone and mostly naked, I waved my trophy triumphantly in the air. I ran to the bed and whispered in Kevin's ear.

"Guess wha-aaat?"

I gently kissed his cheeks, forehead, and neck while he began to stir. He hated being woken in the mornings if he didn't have to be. Jewel, who was also in our bed, laid her head on Kevin's chest.

"We're pregnant!" I burst out, grinning from ear to ear.

"Wow, that was fast! That's so great!" He held his hands victoriously in the air. "I've still got swimmers," he joked, and his arms enveloped me in a bear hug. Jewel pushed her way into our snuggle, ready to share in the excitement. Kevin and I breathed a sigh of relief that we had conceived so quickly. The waiting in between cycles had become the worst part for us. Before we lost multiple pregnancies, the uncertainty or mystery of figuring out our pregnancy status was intriguing. Romantic. Hopeful. But as I wished time away so I could start a new menstrual cycle, it had become an oppressive part of every day. But today was different. Today we had a baby on the way.

It was September, and my mother's birthday is in early October, so I patiently waited to share the exciting news. I knew she wanted desperately to be a grandmother. It was the perfect birthday gift. News of a grandbaby stood in her future! *And really, what are the chances something could go wrong again?* I thought. *Third time's the charm, right?* I figured surely I'd already had my share of bad luck and misfortune. I was again elated to be pregnant, my joy untainted by the other losses, and I felt optimistic about being able to successfully carry this baby. My doctor agreed that despite my previous miscarriages, there was no apparent reason to be concerned.

A few days later I took a break from a work meeting to use the restroom. As soon as I pulled my pants down I couldn't help but notice the pale pink blotches in my underwear. I cursed this omen and wished it away. Sitting right there on the toilet I prayed to a God I wasn't sure was hearing me. I begged Him to let me stay pregnant, to bring this baby into the world, to give me the chance to be a mother. I consciously tried not to overreact. After all, it wasn't an enormous amount of blood. Perhaps it was just some minor spotting. I returned to my meeting and allowed work to occupy my mind. Only an hour later I could feel dampness in my underwear and I returned to the bathroom. All the prayers in the world wouldn't change what was coming next. The bleeding had increased so much that I was forced to stuff toilet paper in my panties until I found an alternative solution. Mindful that I was at work and not wanting to cause a scene, I held my emotions in check. Waddling awkwardly out of the bathroom, I went into my office and called Kevin.

My poor husband. It seemed like I called him only with bad news every time we got pregnant. There were no new words with which to comfort each other. I also spoke to the nurse in Dr. Cohen's office to let them know I was six weeks pregnant but bleeding. Much like the last time, I was told to be prepared for a heavier than usual period. Dr. Cohen insisted I come in for an appointment the following week to discuss next steps. I wrapped up my day and headed home to deal with the disappointment. The drive home felt robotic, surreal. Hadn't I just found out I was pregnant? What could possibly be wrong with me that I lost another one? And so soon?

I couldn't stand being alone in our house, so I grabbed the leash and took Jewel for a long walk. There was a greenway trail just behind our neighborhood. A winding path through the woods, it would provide the temporary escape I needed to absorb my circumstances. My fist clenched the leash as we wandered along. The trees surrounding me stood peaceful in the humidity of the evening. Birds were chirping, the crickets beginning their nightly song. My grip loosened a bit as the animosity toward my situation slowly receded. The woods were so alive with God's creatures. It was a stark contrast to the extinction of life occurring inside me. I marveled in the notion that nature has no bias toward the preservation of life. There was no consideration that I was desperate to have a baby. It was simply not what nature intended. I remembered a college friend who had recently been diagnosed with breast cancer. In spite of her active lifestyle and otherwise clean bill of health, nature didn't take any notice. At only thirty years old, she was preparing for a double mastectomy. None of us was immune to the forces of nature.

I didn't cry about this pregnancy loss until I called my

mother later that night. I'm not sure what was more devastating—my not having a child or my not being able to give her a grandchild. My mother remained positive and supportive in her words, but I was disheartened, beginning to feel defeated. How foolish of me to have expected a good outcome.

"Aren't you two going to have some children?"

"When are you two going to make some babies?"

"What are you two doing in that big house all alone over there? You need to start filling it up!"

"Isn't it about time you start thinking about having some kids?"

"You two would make such good parents. You should really think about having some children."

All were such innocent and seemingly sweet comments from our neighbors and acquaintances, yet all were unintended daggers in my heart. It felt like the harder we tried to make babies and failed, the more the comments came. I realize now, of course, that I was ultrasensitive to anything that was said about babies and family, and the remarks people made were never meant to be hurtful. But as I was literally bleeding from a pregnancy loss, I would have to smile and tolerate the line of questioning. With some friends, I could at least explain that we were trying, or suggest, "It's not always as easy for some couples as it is for others." But that often opened up a conversation that led me to feel I had to explain everything...

and I wasn't sure that emotionally I was ready for that. Talking about it was actually quite therapeutic, but unless the other person had been through a loss like ours, I felt it was hard for him or her to fully relate to our situation. I was frustrated by the casual nature in which people would so easily say, "Oh, don't worry. In time it will happen for you and everything will be all right." They didn't really know that. They couldn't guarantee me a child. Those conversations enraged me rather than comforted me. How dare they suggest they knew everything would be okay, when in reality they had no right to make a promise like that? I had health-care professionals working with me to figure out my losses, and even they weren't so bold as to make that kind of statement. With regard to our closest friends, I suspect they were in an awkward situation. Many were at the same stage in their lives, but successfully having babies. They tried to blend being conscious of and sensitive to our predicament, and yet share the excitement over their own growing families.

The more complicated our fertility story became, the more compassionate I grew toward others, regardless of their struggle. The uneducated but well-intentioned comments from some of our friends made me appreciate that as much as any of us think we can relate to other people's problems, until we walk in their shoes, we really can't understand. Furthermore, I realized Kevin and I were fortunate in that we at least had some health-care coverage for infertility; plus we had some savings that we could put toward it if need be. It was hard to fathom the dilemma faced by some couples who didn't have the financial resources required to even attempt to address their childlessness.

As time passed, the silence in my home became deafening. I often found myself wandering into the room that should have been our nursery. I longed for the cries of a newborn child, the nightly interruptions of a hungry infant needing his milk. Burying my head in my hands, I sometimes crumpled to the floor, alone in my anguish. It didn't help that my hormones were unbalanced. I was usually an even-keeled girl; close friends and my husband would verify that my emotions were fairly kept in check even during that time of the month. But give the most emotionally moderate girl a few pregnancy losses and it's a whole new game. I began to withdraw from customary social outings and retreated to the comfort and privacy of conversations with only my dearest friends. I became someone that at times I didn't recognize, and neither did my husband. Kevin and I began to argue about topics that never would have created a divide between us before. I shot back at him unusually short-tempered remarks and found myself getting angry at trivial things. And rather than respecting my continued drive to get pregnant, Kevin grew irritated with my tenacious behavior. It wasn't that one of us was right and the other of us was wrong. It was just a dilemma neither of us knew how to resolve, and I saw it as more of an urgent problem than Kevin did.

During this time we were not attending any church, and the troubles we experienced only made me more aggravated with a God whose presence I began to doubt. While we tried participating in several churches in our area, we hadn't connected with one in particular. Admittedly, while I began to push God farther away, I still prayed just in case He was listening. I wasn't proud of my spiritual ambiguity. For the first time in my life, my faith was truly faltering, and skepticism about His existence was taking over. Kevin and I were also at quiet odds with each other. In subtle ways he expressed resentment for my perseverance in getting pregnant. I grew worried about the fissure it created in our once rock-solid marriage. I sensed that he conceded to my demands because he felt he had little choice in the matter. While we didn't openly discuss divorce, he knew that walking away from this baby-making goal would by all means lead us down that path.

Despite those apprehensions, my obstinate desire to get pregnant overruled my mounting concern for the health of our marriage. I bounced back from our losses with a resilience that Kevin didn't share. By the time I had my first normal menstrual cycle following our third miscarriage, I was mentally and physically ready to try again. I knew I would need to take the reins. I would need to pursue our next steps, even if it meant I would go about it mostly alone. Kevin, out of pure love for me, and for better or for worse, agreed to try again.

SIX

GIVING MY BODY A BOOST

Kevin and I plugged away and tried to continue our everyday lives with some sense of normalcy. He was better at that than I was. I remained consumed with one ultimate goal: getting pregnant and staying that way for about nine to ten months. Work was very busy for both of us. Luckily it was going well, and we were each entrenched in our careers. I loved the woman I worked for, and she was so understanding of everything Kevin and I had been through. The company was growing by leaps and bounds—we had new accounts, new employees, and the need for additional offices. As the company flourished, I traveled regularly, trying to secure new business or working at meetings for our accounts. Kevin continued to be a top performer for his sales team, growing his existing accounts and acquiring new business in his territory.

I don't believe my pregnancy losses impacted the quality

of my work. It was invaluable to have an employer who I felt "had my back" and was willing to support me and give me a hug or let me have a quiet moment if I needed it. Never once did she challenge me on the doctor appointments that were required with all my bleeding episodes. Not once did she give me a hard time about the extra visits to the ob-gyn office for repeated blood work or ultrasounds.

As the months went on and a vast number of home pregnancy tests were utilized, we toiled to conceive. My menstrual cycle varied dramatically. Some months it was twenty-five days and other months it would be thirty-two days. I felt so exasperated by the unpredictability of it all. I had no idea when to start testing for ovulation, because there was such a difference month-to-month in the length of my cycle. Finally I called Dr. Cohen's office to see whether there was a way to regulate it. After some discussion, we made a plan to put me on Clomid (clomiphene citrate). From what I understood, Clomid is often used as a first line of treatment for infertility, and it helps to induce ovulation. Many physicians resort to Clomid before trying other fertility treatments because it is often the least expensive and least invasive method available. I was informed of the potential side effects, such as vaginal bleeding, breast discomfort, headache, nausea, and vomiting. I was also warned about something called ovarian hyperstimulation syndrome, which included ovarian enlargement, severe gastrointestinal discomfort, shortness of breath, and more. Nevertheless, I felt encouraged to have a course of action to follow. I would be monitored with blood tests and ultrasounds. Because Clomid is an ovulatory stimulant that would force me to release multiple eggs at once, there was an increased chance for me to conceive twins (roughly five to ten percent instead of the usual one percent in the general population) or even triplets (less than one percent chance after taking Clomid). Dr. Cohen said he would recommend that I try the drug for a short time. Prolonged use had been shown to increase the risk of ovarian cancer; if I didn't get pregnant in three months' time, we would move on to another plan.

The first month on the drug I failed to get pregnant. I was devastated. I called Dr. Cohen's office as soon as the pregnancy test was negative and asked for another round of Clomid. He adjusted the timing of my medication, and we tried again. I was reminded to have intercourse every other day during the middle of my cycle. Luckily, Kevin and I were both in town for most of this time and were able to accommodate our designated intercourse schedule. On day twenty-six of my cycle, I woke up early in the morning and took a home pregnancy test. It was a familiar scene. I waited by myself in the bathroom to watch the urine move up the test stick. I was seated on the toilet, feet braced on the cold tile floor, chills creeping up my body. I refused to move, fearful that I could miss the moment when I would see the outcome of our efforts. In the bedroom, both Kevin and Jewel were snoring. While they slept, peacefully unaware of what I was doing, my heart raced in anticipation.

It was positive! Not only that, it was a strong, clearly defined pink line. I immediately wondered whether I was carrying twins. I charged into the bedroom like a racehorse released from her stall and bounded onto our bed, awakening

Kevin. As he turned over to see what had disturbed his dreamy slumber, I waved the test stick in front of him.

"We're pregnant!" I said with total glee. It took him a few seconds to absorb the news, but despite Kevin's trepidations about our journey, he too was genuinely pleased. Kevin, Jewel, and I rearranged ourselves into what we called our family snuggle. Lying there sandwiched between my husband and our pup, I brought the covers up and over us—the blankets shielding us from a world that I knew could take this baby away. I immersed myself in the bliss of the moment.

Dr. Cohen's office performed a blood test to confirm the pregnancy; it indicated that I was pregnant and my hormonal numbers looked strong. Due to my history, my blood levels were monitored closely. For the first couple of months everything progressed normally. As usual, I experienced extreme nausea. It was a welcome symptom that allowed me to appreciate the fact that it meant I was still pregnant. As the weeks passed, tranquillity resumed between Kevin and me. The lead weight resting on our hearts lifted away, leaving space for us to more easily love each other again. We exchanged flirtatious smiles. In the evenings, exhausted from work, we would gather on the couch and settle in for one of our favorite television shows. Kevin would pull me close, tenderly touching my hand or stroking my hair, his affection reassuring me that we would be okay. It was a healthy reprieve from the many months of pressure that once darkened our lives.

For my ten-week checkup, Kevin was able to join me. Given the demands at work, it was an unusual treat to have him there, and we were excited to see our baby on ultrasound.

After the nurse checked my weight and measured my belly, she listened for the baby's heartbeat. *Thump-thump. Thump-thump.* The miraculous sound of life permeated the room. She moved us into the ultrasound room. Dr. Cohen, whom we had grown rather close to by that point, was not in the office that day, so one of his partners in the practice introduced himself to us and began the exam. We could tell he was concerned, but didn't know why at first. Slowly he explained that while the fetus was viable, he was worried because he saw what looked like an edema (collection of fluid) or ascites in the abdomen of the baby. Ascites is fluid that has collected in the peritoneal cavity, which is a gap between the wall of the abdomen and the organs contained within the abdomen. He explained that the accumulation of fluid seen in this area of the baby was not customary. Without getting specific, the doctor cautioned us that this could be very serious. He also expressed concern over what looked like fluid collecting in the brain. While I was not formally educated on the meaning of fluid in either of these areas, I knew enough from my days as a biology major and cancer researcher that this could indeed be a life-threatening problem for a developing fetus. We left the office considering whether there could be a misinterpretation of what the doctor had seen. It was possible he was wrong, or maybe the issue—whatever it was—could resolve itself. We did our best to remain optimistic.

Our instructions were to see a perinatologist later that day at Northside Hospital. In only a few short hours, the specialist was repeating the ultrasound. His conclusion was the same as what we had been told by the obstetrician. The plan was to go back to the ob-gyn office in a week and see whether we still had a viable baby. Kevin and I remained hopeful. Statistically, the odds were in our favor that everything would be fine. We were, after all, already ten weeks pregnant.

While there is some variation in the numbers, we had learned that the odds of having a miscarriage after seeing a heartbeat are low. A fetal heartbeat after eight weeks leads to a 98.5 percent chance your pregnancy will continue; at ten weeks that number rises to 99.3 percent.[1] I was not naive, however, and knew that the odds for miscarriage were higher in women who had a history of recurrent miscarriage. Normal miscarriage rates vary from seventeen to twenty-two percent. But if you have a history of miscarriage, you have a seventeen percent higher chance of having a miscarriage even after seeing a heartbeat on ultrasound.[2] I also learned that only one percent of couples trying to conceive experience three or more consecutive miscarriages.[3] Believe it or not, in those cases, and in particular when there is no history of a live birth, the next pregnancy has a thirty to forty-five percent chance of ending in miscarriage. I fell into that not-so-good category. However, looking at the other side of that figure, it meant I still had a fifty-five to seventy percent chance of delivering a healthy baby.

In the week I waited to return to the ob-gyn's office, I

---

1   Tong S., Kaur, A., Walker, S. P., Bryant, V., Onwude, J. L., Permezel, M. (2008 March). Miscarriage risk for asymptomatic women after a normal first-trimester prenatal visit. *Obstetrics & Gynecology*, 111(3):710-4. doi: 10.1097/ AOG.0b013e318163747c.

2   MD-health.com. (2014 December 8) Miscarriage Chances after Seeing Heartbeat. Retrieved from http://www.md-health.com/Chances-Of-Miscarriage-After-Seeing-Heartbeat.html.

3   Boca Fertility. (2014). Recurrent miscarriages. Retrieved from https://www.bocafertility.com/recurrent_miscarriages.

felt reasonably optimistic about the pregnancy. I was still experiencing severe nausea; plus I didn't have any bleeding or spotting, my expected indication of a pregnancy loss. Kevin and I returned to the ob-gyn office as planned. We sat in the waiting area for nearly an hour. We didn't utter a word to each other. I browsed through magazines, while Kevin read a business article. Multiple times, he put his hand on my thigh in an effort to stop my leg from bouncing up and down. I silently chastised myself for gnawing at the inside of my cheek, a bad nervous habit I had developed in my childhood. Finally, the staff called us into the ultrasound room for our exam. So much hung in the balance. The fate of our child was only minutes away.

I tentatively climbed onto the exam table. If it was good news, I was eager to see and hear more about our baby. If it was bad news, I wanted to rewind and not go through with the exam, as if never having the ultrasound would undo our circumstances. I knew that was foolish, but desperation was taking my mind down an imaginary path where only a good outcome was possible. If I didn't see a dead baby, then I wouldn't have a dead baby.

Dr. Cohen gave us a tender greeting, and Kevin held my hand as the doctor lifted my shirt and spread warm ultrasound gel across my abdomen. Knowing what was at stake, he focused all his attention on the ultrasound screen. He quickly found the baby's heart and looked at me with regret. This may not have been his baby, but it was obvious that he felt our pain in this moment. It was one of the things I liked best about him

—his compassion for his patients was palpable. He took my hand in his and looked at the two of us.

"I'm so sorry. The baby no longer has a heartbeat." At eleven weeks' gestation, we had lost our fourth baby. Kevin squeezed my hand tighter and leaned down to embrace me. I felt so foolish for being hopeful. I should have learned to expect the worst. That was my norm. *Really, God? Again? Why does this keep happening to us?* All those hopes and dreams for yet another baby were gone in an instant. What were God's intentions for us? I certainly didn't place trust in Him at this point. It seemed that when I needed God the most He was letting me down. What lesson could I possibly be learning from these losses?

My heart beat with an empty ache. There was a fragile tension between my wanting to believe in God—needing to believe in a God who loved me—and giving up on my belief altogether that a higher power even existed. I was desperate to escape the pain that pursued me. No matter what attempts I made to run from it, pain found me and pulled me to the ground, beating me senseless when I was already down. Anguish seeped deep into the core of my body and flowed through me, leaving holes everywhere. The once abundant joy in me was displaced by the indescribable agony of losing a child. When would joy ever find its way back into me again? And what about grace or peace? Could they navigate their way through the puzzle I had become? Could they fill in some of the missing pieces?

I said a silent prayer that I would repeat many times over in the months that followed:

Heavenly Father,

You have blessed me in so many ways. You have surrounded me with wonderful people, a supportive and loving family, amazing friends. You've given me skills that enrich my life and allow me to give back to those around me. But please, God, please help me understand—why did you make me good at making angels?

I looked up at Dr. Cohen. "What's the plan next?" I asked as I held back tears. It was time to yet again pick up the pieces and figure out how to move on. I refused to take the time to grieve. Adversity would not win this battle. I wanted a baby, and fussing about the one we had just lost wasn't going to get me to the next step any sooner.

I was scheduled for a D&C (dilation and curettage) the following day. One of the things that made this loss different is that we were able to test some tissue that was taken from the baby during the procedure. It indicated that the baby had Turner syndrome, which at least gave us an explanation for the loss.

It was, for the first and only time in all of our pregnancy losses, the one "legitimate" or explicable reason we ever lost a baby. From what I understand, Turner is a chromosomal abnormality in which all or part of one of the sex chromosomes is absent. It was explained to me that ninety-nine percent of Turner syndrome conceptions end in spontaneous abortion (like this one) or stillbirth. It was "nature's way" of handling an unhealthy baby, which at least made sense to me

—this particular child was not meant to be. While a very low percentage of babies can survive with Turner, I suspect there are varying degrees of severity of the disease. This baby, like most with Turner, did not make it to full term.

Only a day or so after the loss of that baby, I was back at work. I was sitting at my desk when I suddenly felt severe cramping and a strange oozing feeling coming from my crotch. I rushed to the bathroom. I pulled down my pants and was shocked to see enormous clots on the thick pad that was supposed to help with heavy bleeding after a D&C. This was by no means ordinary. The clots ranged in size from golf balls to tennis balls; it was hard for me to believe what I saw. I had heard of hemorrhaging like this, but was astounded it was happening to me. *Isn't losing the baby enough? Why are so many things going wrong? Why does this keep happening to me?*

Amid my fear of passing out, I calmly cleaned up the mess in the bathroom and made my way to my boss's office. Concerned with the amount of blood loss, I didn't think I should be alone. It was getting to be late in the evening, and I wanted to be sure someone at the office knew my condition. My boss brought me water and a snack, which I quickly consumed. I called Dr. Cohen's office and got no answer; the phones had been switched to their answering service. I was only a few minutes from his office. Feeling more confident that I would not faint, I decided to drive by and see whether there was any staff wrapping up their day. On the way to the ob-gyn I called Kevin and left him a message. I knew he was in a surgical procedure and unavailable to help me with this minicrisis.

I knocked hard on the glass door of the practice until a receptionist in the far back heard me. I explained what was going on and asked whether Dr. Cohen could see me. Fortunately she allowed me in, and he came into the exam room as soon as he was available. In his usual sweet and comforting tone, he spoke to me about what was going on. He also examined me to be sure I was not at risk for some other incident. It was just my bad luck…another strike against me and my body in my attempt to get pregnant and carry a baby to term. Hemorrhaging, as it turns out, is one of the possible risks and complications associated with a D&C. I needed to grin and bear it, and make my way through this as I had all the other obstacles we'd faced thus far. Over the next few days, I was closely monitored by Dr. Cohen, and the hemorrhaging ceased quite rapidly after the one memorable episode at work.

SEVEN

TO BE OR NOT TO BE

After that last loss, we sat down with Dr. Cohen for a strategy session. He informed us that it was time to move on to a fertility specialist—one who would help us improve our chances of having a healthy baby. Dr. Cohen didn't necessarily feel at this point that there was anything "wrong" with either one of us…but given the number of losses we'd had and the circumstances, it was time to take a different approach.

On one hand it worried me that our case was bad enough that I should need to see a reproductive endocrinologist (a doctor who treats infertility). On the other hand it was like music to my ears. Besides the two-month worry-free break we'd had during the last pregnancy, Kevin and I had been experiencing a rough patch in our marriage, and I was beginning to lose hope that we would ever be able to have a child. The strain on us to always be working on making a baby had not been easy. The physical and logistical requirements were cumbersome in light of our schedules, and I had a difficult time feeling relaxed about pretty much anything. When anyone asked how I was, I often gave a completely fake answer, which only made me more irritated. I knew nobody really wanted to hear how upset I was over our infertility troubles, but by the same token, it was exhausting to lie about my state of mind. So many of my friends were easily having babies, and I fought an internal battle between being happy for them and being envious of their situation. I was not proud of that. I felt ashamed to even think of wishing they could empathize with me. I knew that would mean they too would have lost a pregnancy, or not been able to conceive, or experienced any other number of infertility problems. I didn't actually wish those atrocities on anyone, but I admit that I did desire that my friends knew and better understood how I felt.

The misery Kevin and I had been through combined with the uncertainty about children in our future put our marriage in a constant state of tension. We were fortunate to love each other unconditionally, and we vowed to get through this obstacle together. Divorce was never once even discussed, despite the fact that at times it may have seemed easier to walk away from each other. Even so, I sometimes wondered whether our relationship would implode over this one predicament in our lives. My persistence in seeking a solution to our child-bearing dilemma was a stark contrast to what became Kevin's willingness to abandon the idea altogether. We tolerated each other's position just enough and had compassion for what the other person felt. I didn't hate him for feeling like we should consider being a family as just the two of us, for thinking that perhaps we should give up on the whole idea of having a child. It was understandable after losing four babies. But I was resentful that he didn't share my enthusiasm despite our struggle. I towed the weight for both of us when it came to finding a solution. I was the one who set up all the doctor appointments. I was the one keeping track of my hormone cycle and peeing on sticks most mornings of the month. I was the one getting my blood drawn every couple days. I was the one getting nauseous and vomiting for months. I was the one bleeding for weeks or getting a D&E/D&C when we lost a baby. I was the one whose hormones were toying with my emotions. I was the one who was getting older and less fertile by the second. I was the one whose body was failing our children.

In my opinion, by comparison, he had the easy part of the job.

And then I would realize how much focus was put on what "I" wanted and not what "we" wanted. His lack of enthusiasm wasn't meant to diminish the fact that he wanted children. He just didn't have quite the same agenda as I did in terms of timing or drive to get it done quickly. The scheduled sex, my short-temperedness, the pressure from me to try again, the heartache and disappointment every time we lost a baby, the anger and frustration that followed each loss—he was exhausted by it all. I knew that if he could, he would have taken some of the burden off of me and put it on himself.

As far as our faith was concerned, God was essentially absent in our lives. I was too wrapped up in worrying about what I wanted instead of what was meant to be. I had no ability to consider that perhaps God had a greater purpose for me in this journey to make a family. My self-absorption pushed Him out rather than turning me toward Him and helping me rely on Him alone for the answer. I was ashamed for questioning my relationship with God, but by the same token, I was too hurt to understand that perhaps the pain was intentional—a part of His divine plan for me.

At this point, together Kevin and I began to search for a renewed faith and a plan of action to bring a baby into our lives. We were completely open to the idea of having children by any means, whether that meant they were biologically ours or not. That left us with several options. I had tackled, and conquered, problems in many other aspects of my life thus far. Surely there had to be a solution to this devastating hardship.

Dr. Cohen was thorough in his evaluation of why I was having trouble carrying. He evaluated my blood, sent me for a hysterosalpingogram (an X-ray that examines the inside of the uterus, fallopian tubes, and surrounding area), and performed all the other first steps that might indicate where in my reproductive system we were encountering a problem. I had proven I could readily conceive (even if it took a few months), and maybe all I needed was the right embryo. Perhaps having a baby could be easy for us with a little bit of assistance? By the time Dr. Cohen advised us to get a consultation from an infertility specialist, we were ready to embrace the idea and felt encouraged to move forward.

Almost immediately I scheduled an appointment with Dr. Joseph Goldsmith, who worked for a very reputable infertility clinic in Atlanta, Georgia. Kevin and I arrived right on time for our appointment. A sign on the registration desk read, "If your wait is longer than 10 minutes, please let the receptionist know." A smile emerged from my lips. I liked this place already. They totally understood—those of us who were here had spent months, or maybe even years waiting to have a baby. The last thing we wanted was more waiting. The receptionist greeted us and assured us the doctor would be with us shortly.

Kevin and I spent an hour in our first consultation with Dr. Goldsmith simply reviewing our history and talking about a plan. We discovered that Dr. Goldsmith was a man who spoke bluntly. His straightforward approach appealed to Kevin and me, because we needed to know the truth in order to move on to whatever next step was ahead. Time was of the essence. Like Dr. Cohen, Dr. Goldsmith had a good sense of humor, and every now and then he would poke fun at various elements of the infertility process in order to lighten the mood. This didn't detract from the serious topic at hand; it just allowed us to relax a bit.

Dr. Goldsmith concluded our discussion by informing us, with a good sense of confidence, that he could help us have a baby. He came up with a plan for me to begin with self-administered injections of a hormone (follicle-stimulating hormone, or FSH) that would increase my egg production, followed by intrauterine insemination (IUI). I was a good candidate for IUI because it often is used for people with unexplained infertility problems. In simple terms, IUI involves putting sperm inside a woman's uterus to facilitate fertilization and increase the chances that healthy sperm will reach and fertilize the egg on their own. It is a less expensive and less invasive option compared to in vitro fertilization (IVF). He explained that early in my menstrual cycle I would administer the FSH. Then, around the time of ovulation, sperm that was previously collected and washed would be inserted directly into my uterus via a catheter. It would be a procedure that maximized the number of sperm cells getting to my eggs, and would require minimal discomfort. This plan would assist my body in what it could already do naturally, but would optimize my chances of conception with a healthy embryo.

I felt emboldened by this newfound idea. I walked out of there a happy lady. A lady with a plan. Sometimes that's all it takes to keep me going.

Kevin and I were thoroughly rescreened for any medical or physical abnormalities that could be causing our fertility issues. Dr. Cohen had already performed a number of these tests, but several of them needed repeating, given our multiple pregnancy losses and the time that had passed since the tests were performed. As anticipated, everything appeared physically normal for both of us.

During one of our prescreening medical-workup visits, I needed to have a transvaginal ultrasound (transvaginal meaning "through the vagina") to make sure my uterus was clear and healthy. I had experienced transvaginal ultrasounds plenty of times before. In general, the technique is a pelvic ultrasound used to examine the reproductive organs. During the many pregnancies and procedures of my past, the early checkups or examinations always included one. Transvaginal ultrasounds were a more accurate way to check the fetal heartbeat, measure my cervix, examine the placenta, check for cysts or fibroids, evaluate unexplained bleeding, and more. On this day, Kevin was in the room with me. The tech was preparing to insert the extralong ultrasound wand into me. Though he'd been with me before, Kevin had never noticed the size of the wand, and it caught him off guard. He watched with fascination as she unrolled a condom onto it.

"Wow, that could make a man feel insignificant," he said with a grin on his face. Kevin's sense of humor is to share with all, rather than keeping things to himself, even at times like this.

And kudos to the technician holding the wand, who without pause fired back at him, "A woman earlier today told me this was the best thing she's had all month!" I laughed out loud at that, and paused for a moment, relating to that poor woman and her husband—in reality, they were probably exhausted from all their procreative efforts and didn't have the energy for "sex without a cause," if they had a desire for any sex at all. The only action she had probably seen lately was from the ultrasound wand. In all probability she was in the middle of an IVF cycle, where intercourse wasn't required to get pregnant.

The patient's comment resonated with me. It seemed like forever since Kevin and I had an appetite for spontaneous sex brimming with lust and romance. Rather than making love, the intimacy in our relationship was about making babies. As a couple, we already faced the challenge of busy travel schedules related to our work. Add to that four pregnancy losses, weeks of ancillary bleeding, and the dynamics of infertility—saying it had impacted our sexuality was a sobering understatement. For me, it was a difficult transition from a medical procedure where five or six people were walking into the room—my feet secured in stirrups and legs wide-open with all my private parts on display—to feeling sexy with my husband. My sexual organs were constantly under scrutiny for their failure to work properly. When making love, all I could think about was whether we were conceiving, putting a serious damper on the enjoyment level for me, and also for Kevin. In fact, the act itself served only to remind me that we were struggling to have a baby. For Kevin, performing intercourse on demand in the bedroom couldn't have been easy. And basically, regardless of the path we took under the guidance of an infertility specialist, Kevin would need to ejaculate in a cup. Surely that wasn't an activity he felt excited to do. For some people, a depressed libido might have been from fertility drugs or other medication. In our case, neither of us was on medication. We knew the deterioration of our sex life was purely a psychological side effect during this phase of our marriage.

During my next visit to the infertility clinic, I quickly learned how to give myself the injections, and was monitored closely on ultrasound for follicle (egg) production. Luckily, all those years of lab research paid off, as I had no fear of needles. They would adjust my FSH dose according to what they saw on the ultrasound. I was warned that I might become moody, but to be honest, I don't think it affected me at all, and Kevin agreed.

In the meantime, Kevin was notified of *his* responsibilities. They would need to collect a sperm sample from him for testing, as well as get fresh samples from him at the end of the IUI process on the insemination days.

Dr. Goldsmith informed him, "You will need to 'make love to Tupperware,' as I like to call it. You can either provide a sample at home that could quickly be brought into the office for processing, or you can utilize the facilities at our clinic."

He then went on with something of a pep talk: "This is the part of our consult I know men say they have a hard time with. They try to tell me it's not something they can do, or claim they are not comfortable with it, or they just can't make it happen. I get lots of excuses."

Kevin cut him off. "I've got it covered, Doc. Just give me some time alone so I can get on with it and take care of business. Then we can both go on with our day."

With a grin, Dr. Goldsmith responded, "Finally, a man who can tell it like it is."

It was December 30, 2002. The night before the intrauterine insemination, I had to have a deeper injection into my butt that required someone else give me the shot. I recruited Kevin for the job. It seemed only fair that he participate in the workup of our future baby. Up until this point, for the most part I had acted alone in this process. My days and weeks were consumed with regular injections and/or ultrasounds. Besides his crucial sperm donation, Kevin was not heavily involved.

Given my petite frame, I begged the nurse to provide us with a shorter needle than the one they normally use for intramuscular injections (the regular needle looked *huge* compared to my little body). Fortunately she agreed. Kevin still gawked at the sight of it. This shot would deliver medication to stimulate my ovulation. It was crucial that we got it right.

That evening, we got ourselves primed for the injection. Oddly enough, we convened in our kitchen. The shot needed to take place at a particular time, and Kevin had just walked in the door from work, pressing to make it home in time for the scheduled appointment with each other. I closed the blinds on nearby windows, pulled my pants down, and looked at him over my shoulder. "Put the needle in quickly, without hesitation, or it will hurt," I told him, just as the nurse had instructed. Offering a demonstration, I held my thumb, index finger, and middle finger together so he could see that he was supposed to hold the syringe like a dart. I turned back around and braced myself on the counter in front of me, gripping it with both hands. Without warning, Kevin jabbed me with the needle.

Believe it or not, I barely felt it! Just a teeny pinch. *That wasn't so bad. Well worth all these shots to make a baby.* I congratulated Kevin on a job well-done and proceeded to make our dinner.

The next day was New Year's Eve. I walked into the infertility office carrying the little brown baggie that had been provided. It contained Kevin's fresh sperm sample. I sat there holding it, waiting to be called. There were others in the waiting room clutching their little brown baggies too. It was precious cargo. A while later, the doctor on call that day performed my IUI. I was on the exam table, hips elevated, and a simple procedure to insert the sperm was all it took.

I felt like saying, "Seriously, that's it?" but knew that would sound foolish. They wanted me to remain with my hips elevated for twenty minutes, and then I would be allowed to go home and spend the remainder of the day resting quietly. I pondered the thought that Kevin hadn't even been in the room for the potential conception of our child. His caseload at work was demanding, and due to the nature of the process (my insemination day was a bit of a moving target), it wasn't entirely easy for him to join me. While I would have preferred that he be there, I felt I had been demanding in so many other respects that I didn't push him to come with me.

The past few days I had started feeling a little bloated, but that night I felt horribly crampy and uncomfortable. I diverted my attention to dreams of our future child. The following morning I awoke to repeat the insemination process one more time. It was New Year's Day, 2003. The chance to make a baby again.

Kevin told me he planned to remain at home, and this time I was offended by his lack of participation. I could under-stand that he preferred to collect his sample in the privacy of our own house, but he could have come to the appointment with me. The least he could do was be there to hold my hand or show me his support. It was a holiday, and today he had no work excuse. The insemination wouldn't take long and he knew that. I choked back tears as I pretended to be fine with his decision. That was not uncommon in our marriage at the time. Rather than pushing back on something that frustrated either one of us, we just gave in or ignored the other person's feelings.

I struggled to understand why he wasn't more engaged in the making of our baby. I wondered whether he resisted participating in events like the insemination as a stubborn way to indicate that he was not as eager as I was to move forward with our plans. There was certainly a degree of resentment from both of us. On plenty of nights over the past year I had lain in bed quietly crying myself to sleep, tortured by our multiple miscarriages. Kevin was unaware of those episodes, completely tuned out of my emotional status. That, or he pretended he didn't know. I married a man who had little tolerance for crying and emotional chaos. Which is why I didn't lean on him for comfort on those dreadful, pain-filled nights, when the pregnancy losses we had endured sometimes felt like too much to bear. I harbored a lot of anger toward him for lacking the ability to see (or act on) how upset I was. We were supposed to be a team.

I made the conscious decision to hold off on speaking to him about not coming to the insemination. From experience, I knew it was best for both of us not to argue a point in the heat of the moment. I needed to let my emotions settle down, get to my appointment, and make a baby—with or without him there.

I headed into the doctor's office with my little brown baggie, feeling less embarrassed having done this once before, and knowing everyone else in the office was there for the same reason. They didn't care. We all had the same goal in mind: We were all in different phases of trying to make babies. No one was laughing at me for toting what looked like a lunch sack, filled with sperm.

The procedure was an exact repeat from the day before. I returned home to spend the afternoon resting on the couch. I was terribly uncomfortable for the remainder of the day and through the night. My belly was extremely distended, and I had some of the most severe abdominal pain I've ever experienced. I didn't remember being told it could be so bad. The next few days I took it easy and allowed myself to physically lie low. The New Year's holiday was perfect, as it gave me some additional recovery time before I returned to work.

Early in the morning only ten days after the IUI was complete, I woke up with a slight twinge of nausea. My gut told me this was a good thing. I bolted to the bathroom, grabbed my pregnancy test stick, and sat on the toilet. I began to pee. *Please be positive; please be positive.*

I didn't move from the seat as I watched the urine move up the stick. A barely visible pink line appeared past the control line. It was positive! Seated on the bathroom throne, I shook my body around in a happy dance. I remained there and just stared at the test over and over again. *Thank you, God. Thank you, Dr. Goldsmith.* Even though this was my fifth pregnancy, seeing a positive result was like winning the lottery —it could never get old. I finally got up from the toilet and placed the test stick on the counter near Kevin's sink, leaving the evidence for him to find later. He was on the road for work, so I crawled back into bed and called him to announce our good news. We shared a cautiously optimistic attitude, but because of the IUI process, we felt more comfortable than usual that this pregnancy would be successful. Plus, it was an emotional and financial relief to have a positive pregnancy test after only one month of trying. I hung up the phone and called Jewel into our bed. She happily obliged and nosed her way deep under the covers. I scooted my way down to her and held her face in my hands.

"You're going to be a big sister, sweet girl!" Jewel had been my child up until now, and I considered her part of the family. Sensing my excitement, she wet my face with a sloppy kiss from my chin up to my forehead. We snuggled for a while until I finally made my way into the shower to start getting ready for work.

My scheduled blood test at Dr. Goldsmith's office wasn't for another day or two, but I knew the answer already. My increasing nausea confirmed it for me. I was pregnant. I tentatively wondered how many babies we had conceived. When doing IUI, you do have an increased chance of having multiples. I had some concern about that, only because of my small stature and the number of miscarriages I had already endured.

A couple days later, my blood work confirmed a positive pregnancy result.

In the next few days, Dr. Goldsmith's lab regularly repeated my blood work to evaluate the quantitative amount of beta hCG levels in my system. Human chorionic gonadotropin is the hormone produced by cells that form the placenta following implantation of the embryo. In normal pregnancies, hCG levels double roughly every forty-eight to seventy-two hours. In my case, the doctor quickly discovered they were not increasing normally. In addition, I had begun spotting the smallest bit. Traces of pale pink colored my underwear. It was different from the spotting or streaks I had seen in other pregnancy losses, so I remained calm for now, satisfied that I was being carefully monitored by my doctor.

Then the nurse phoned me to tell me there was a problem with the numbers they saw in my blood work, and we needed to meet with Dr. Goldsmith right away. I informed her of the spotting and our appointment was scheduled for the following day.

Dr. Goldsmith was known for being very direct, not the warm-and-fuzzy type. He doesn't waste anyone's time at a point when time is precious. Despite his usual sense of humor, there was no laughter on this matter. As was becoming customary for us, our joy in celebrating a healthy pregnancy was short-lived.

He sat us down and began discussing his concerns about the blood work reports. He explained the reasons this pregnancy would not be a viable one. With every new pregnancy we were offered a glimmer of hope, and we would feel lifted up, only to have that pregnancy falter a short time later. I prepared for the worst as Dr. Goldsmith continued the consultation.

Challenging him, I interrupted. "Dr. Goldsmith, I have a scientific background and I spent years in the lab doing research. I need you to give me some real numbers. How sure are you that we are going to lose this baby?"

He paused and looked at us regretfully. "Stacey, I am

ninety-nine-point-nine percent sure you are not having this baby. This is what the statistics say based on your hCG numbers," he said, quoting the research data. "I know it's very disappointing. If I'm wrong, I'll eat my hat."

"How often have you ever been wrong?" I asked. I knew the practice of medicine was an art, not a black-and-white science.

"In all my years of practice I have been wrong on this matter only once before. You know, when the mother had that baby she brought me a cake in the shape of a hat. I wish I could be wrong in this way more often, but I'm telling you this based on everything we know. According to your numbers you will not be having this baby. I'm really sorry."

I had heard that before, and I appreciated his honesty. Only this time things were slightly different. This baby wasn't dead yet.

Because the developing embryo wasn't far enough along for him to even detect a heartbeat, there wasn't the medical ability to confirm or deny the viability of the baby. The suggestion was that if we wanted to move things along faster, we could use methotrexate to clear the supposedly nonviable embryonic tissue from my body in order to attempt another IUI cycle faster.

There was something in me that refused to accept what I was being told. Despite all the losses we had endured, I didn't consider this baby gone until I knew we were truly without a living embryo. I would fight for this child until the end. That was the least I could do for our baby. Kevin agreed with me wholeheartedly. We decided before we even left Dr. Goldsmith's office that day that I would not take the methotrexate. If God meant for us to lose this baby we would wait for it to happen, regardless of the scientific data. In addition, my body had been through so many procedures, both in evaluating my fertility and in losing previous pregnancies, that we felt it was best for nature to take its course.

And so we waited.

At five and a half weeks I went in for an ultrasound, and there was a heartbeat. Statistically it didn't make sense. I continued to experience light bleeding for the next two and a half weeks.

Later, at about eight weeks' gestation, when I had another ultrasound, there were limb buds, and other normal anatomical developments. The all-consuming nausea I started feeling immediately upon discovering I was pregnant never subsided. At every checkup, the baby showed progress just as he/she should, but was always smaller than he/she should be (about a week in size smaller than usual). My hCG levels never normalized, registering well below the expected levels. Nobody could explain it. Nature, and what we saw on the ultrasound screen, was not following the scientific data. It was an emotionally bizarre time for us. We wavered between excitement on one hand that things were progressing, and on the other hand keeping our guard up, knowing that the status of our pregnancy could change at any time. We divulged the news to our families and prepared them for an uncertain outcome. At the end of each day, I said a prayer of gratitude that we retained the pregnancy.

Finally, at the three-month mark, Dr. Goldsmith called

us for his final consult. My bleeding had stopped, the baby was growing, and we had ceased trying to track or explain my hCG numbers. The baby was measuring small but developing normally. I had a nuchal translucency study at about twelve weeks. An NT screening, which involves an ultrasound performed by a perinatologist, can help give parents-to-be a better idea of the risk associated with a fetus as it relates to Down syndrome, several other chromosomal disorders, and congenital heart defects. The data from the ultrasound is combined with some specific blood tests to serve as a predictor for those concerns. For us, it was a safer way to have some indication as to the health of our baby than a more invasive alternative to genetic testing. Given my past miscarriages, it was not ideal for me to have an amniocentesis, for instance, or even genetic analysis from chorionic villus sampling. Both of those techniques were associated with an increased risk of miscarriage. While the results of the NT screening could not give us absolute certainty about the good health of our baby, we were satisfied that our fetus was unlikely to have any of the chromosomal/heart problems they were looking to find.

While the future of this baby was still somewhat uncertain, Dr. Goldsmith happily released me into the care of my ob-gyn, Dr. Cohen, for regular obstetrical care. My veins were grateful as well—my arms had become rather bruised from the frequent intravenous blood tests. With a warm hug from Dr. Goldsmith and a hopeful outlook, we were off!

I remained quiet about my pregnancy for another month or so, cautious about bringing others on this emotional roller-coaster ride with us. I informed colleagues at work at about sixteen weeks' gestation. It felt good to be able to reveal how nauseated I had been feeling, which sometimes impacted me during work meetings. I also could no longer conceal my ever-growing belly. Loose clothes can work only so long before maternity clothes become a requirement, especially on a petite frame. I treasured the act of shopping for a few work-appropriate maternity outfits.

I was elated. Overjoyed. Euphoric. I was thoroughly taking delight in being pregnant. Most of my worries faded, as it seemed like things would be favorable this time.

By contrast, although Kevin was thrilled with the idea of a baby on the way, he was careful to temper his enthusiasm. The uncertainty of why we had lost three of the four previous pregnancies left Kevin feeling as though we could not ignore the risks going forward.

Every time he received an unexpected phone call from me he would hesitate before picking up the phone, bracing himself for the news of another pregnancy loss. Apprehension resided in him, and prevented him from feeling truly relaxed and at ease even with this pregnancy.

We found out on one of the early ultrasounds that I was carrying a baby boy. When I was a child, I always expected to be a mother who wanted the gender of my children to remain a mystery until birth. Well, my opinion on the subject had changed. We had so many negative surprises and countless unknowns in our pregnancies that it gave us some additional exuberance to be able to better identify with the baby by knowing its gender. Add to that the fact that we lost four other babies without knowing their sex, and every positive data point was somehow comforting.

Quite honestly, at this point Kevin and I had seen so many ultrasounds that we could nearly read them ourselves. We predicted that it was a boy when the ultrasound tech got to that area of the anatomy. We glanced her way for formal confirmation. Kevin was thrilled, and I was happy too. It really didn't matter to us. Just a full-term, healthy child—that was all we were asking for.

At about eighteen to twenty weeks my nausea finally subsided and I really started feeling good. I was getting my energy back and I had an appetite again. In all of my pregnancies I always had severe nausea, and why doctors call it "morning sickness" befuddles me. I was nauseated morning, noon, and night. And it didn't go away until well into the second trimester. Yet I adored being pregnant and I would do it all again in an instant if I could.

Kevin always laughs and says that God got it right when he made women the bearer of children. "If men had to reproduce we would go extinct. Imagine a bunch of guys sitting around a bar while one of them talks about all of the physical changes he went through during and after the pregnancy, stretching and tearing just to name a few!" He would continue: "The other guys would sit there and cringe, saying, 'There's no way I'm doing that!'"

Kevin admits that most men wouldn't easily tolerate the nine to ten months leading up to childbirth and the monthly menstrual cycles females have to endure from puberty. God did get it right. He then added, "Consider that some women have babies, and a little while later, despite tearing from perineum to anus, they want to have another one." As I contemplated his theory I wondered whether, in the back of their minds, men were questioning the sanity of women. In many cases one could argue that women inherit an unstoppable, relentless drive to have children.

In all fairness, Kevin has always said that being a spectator during all of our losses and procedures was the hardest part for him. While logically he knew he couldn't relieve me of the emotional pain, he certainly wished he could replace me on the exam table and bear the brunt of all the physical pain and hardship I had to go through. Maybe he felt he was physically and emotionally stronger than I was, or maybe he just felt it would be easier for him to tolerate the pain rather than watch helplessly as I went through it.

On a Saturday morning, just shy of twenty-four weeks' gestation, I went to the bathroom and discovered I was bleeding. I didn't become hysterical. I knew occasional spotting could occur in pregnancy; I had bled worse during the first three weeks of this one. Fortunately this was a small amount of blood. I phoned the doctor on call for my ob-gyn office. Given my long and complicated history, he instructed me to go to the emergency room. Kevin drove me there as we engaged in casual conversation. We attempted to pretend this was a routine visit, operating under the assumption that the baby was fine. I was seen quickly by the emergency room staff. They hooked me up to a fetal heart-rate monitor and performed a pelvic exam. I took deep breaths, reminding myself to remain calm, which was easier for me to do during this period of uncertainty because I could see the baby's heartbeat on the monitor. There were no signs of distress, and the doctor's exam led him to believe there was no real cause for concern. In short, after hours of evaluation, everything looked normal. They released me that day and things seemed fine. The bleeding stopped by that evening.

I went back to work on Monday as usual, but decided to call Dr. Cohen and inform him of the weekend's events. I explained that I was scheduled to fly out of town for business on Tuesday. He insisted that I come in for an appointment that day. I did not have permission to leave town until I saw him.

Later that day, as I was lying on the exam table—a place that had begun to feel like my second home—Dr. Cohen asked, "Have you been having any contractions?"

"No, I don't think so," I said cautiously.

"Well, you, my dear, will be driving straight to the hospital. Do not stop at work. Do not go home to get things. I want you to drive straight to Northside Hospital and check yourself in immediately. Starting now you are on strict bed rest. I will call and make all the necessary arrangements so they expect your arrival. You will be spending the next few weeks in the hospital until we get you far enough along that we can discuss the next step."

I was speechless. Perhaps it was a good thing I was already lying down.

He explained further: "Your cervix is dilated and effaced. You could go into labor and have this baby soon if we are not very, very careful and cautious. You will not be doing much of anything for at least the next few weeks, and probably for the remainder of your pregnancy."

Stunned and in complete disbelief, I drove myself to the hospital.

EIGHT

THE MOM BRIGADE

I called Kevin to let him know the news, but needed to leave a message, since he was in a case. It had all been going so well. *This baby has already proven to be a miracle from the start, and now this? Can't we catch a break somewhere?* Remembering Dr. Cohen's warning about proceeding directly to the hospital, I called my boss next. Dumbfounded by what I had been told, I was unsure what to tell her as it related to work. I didn't know when I could return to the office, or even whether I would be allowed to leave the hospital until the baby was born. We decided to give it a few days and see what direction things were going.

Before I left Dr. Cohen's office, I made one last crucial phone call—to my mother. I explained the situation to her and, God bless her, she said she would come right away to help. I expected her to pack a minimal amount and come stay for a few days until we figured out a plan to manage things.

When Kevin got the news of my prescribed hospital stay, he was two and a half hours away with a customer in south Georgia. Clearly concerned for the well-being of both the baby and me, he called me back from the operating room as soon as he heard the message. The doctor he was working with did not appreciate Kevin stepping away from the case. Kevin was always the consummate professional.

As Kevin walked back toward the surgical field the physician stood motionless with his head turned toward him. He quipped sternly, "Do you have a more pressing matter to tend to?"

Kevin explained to the doctor that I had been admitted to the hospital. The doctor happened to know we had lost several other pregnancies and quickly changed his tune, encouraging him to leave immediately. Kevin rushed to get home; he planned to pack some things I had requested he bring to the hospital.

While at home getting my items ready, Kevin heard a car door slam. Peeking through the blinds, he could see the driveway from our master bedroom window. Much to his surprise, he realized my mother had arrived. With a frantic look on her face, she opened up the trunk of her minivan. It took all of her strength to unload a gargantuan suitcase from the back of the car.

In that moment, he had a sense of both relief that help was on the way, and utter concern that my mother was moving in for the long haul.

It was clear from the size of the suitcase that she had packed for a month. She was here to stay for the duration. She knew Kevin was on the road constantly, and I would need help at home. I suspect she also wanted to be near me and ready to get to the hospital quickly in case things got a little tougher. We had no idea how long or difficult this ordeal might get. I figured we would need to board our dog, Jewel, but with my mother staying at our house, that would be taken care of too. She could water plants, gather our mail, handle groceries, laundry, etc. She stepped up big-time, and we will forever be grateful. Not many families are lucky enough to have a mother, friend, or relative so giving and capable (and also so available). We hit the jackpot. For me, there was nothing quite like having my own mother care for me at a time like this.

At twenty-four weeks' gestation, my bed-rest journey began. When I got to the hospital, the staff was fully prepared and immediately took me to a room. I was hooked up to monitors of all kinds—a fetal monitor, blood-pressure machine, heart-rate monitor. Later that same day I started having fairly severe contractions that I could easily identify. Luckily I had them after I was admitted to the hospital, so it was simple to monitor how steadily they came on. The other blessing in our lives that day was Dr. Cohen and his persistence in sending me to the hospital. We remain eternally grateful for the relentless care and compassion he showed in making that decision.

I was given bed-rest instructions as follows:

- You must lie completely flat all day long.

- You are permitted to sit up only twenty minutes a day.

- You may shower once every three days. Maybe. We'll see how your cervix looks and give you permission based on that.

- This one should be obvious, but you may not be intimate in any way with your husband. Absolutely no hanky-panky.

For the next three weeks I was closely managed by the staff of the high-risk perinatal unit at Northside Hospital. It was hard to find a moment of silence.

During my hospital stay and for the remainder of my pregnancy I had contractions *every few minutes*. They literally did not stop for any substantial length of time. Based on my strict limitations, I described bed rest to my friends as "ten toes up, not yet six feet under."

My contractions were controlled with an oral drug called terbutaline, a tocolytic agent. My understanding is that doctors prescribe it to suppress or delay preterm labor because it inhibits contractions of myometrial smooth muscle cells in the uterus, giving it the ability to slow or even prevent contractions. We hoped it would keep me from going into full-blown labor. I quickly learned to turn to my left side, which helped maximize the blood flow to my uterus during the contractions. When I went to sleep at night, I tried to fall asleep on that side to get a better night's sleep and help the baby as much as possible. Nurses would wake me every few hours to check all my vitals, and to check the baby too. To say the least, I did not have one good night of deep or restful sleep. I did, however, appreciate the intense care I was given. Having all those contractions at home would have been nerve-racking.

I had every incentive to do as well as I could. Unlike other patients who may be incapable of moving for long periods of time, my bed rest had a distinct goal: one healthy baby boy. I instantly set my mind to the task at hand. If this was what it was going to take for me to carry a full-term baby, then so be it. Great patience would lead to a great reward.

At this point, I'm sure my husband wondered when he would ever have regular, spontaneous sex with me again. Between the months of scheduled sex during ovulation, the early onset of nausea once I was pregnant, the bleeding episodes during pregnancy, the bleeding from loss of pregnancy or surgery, and now prescribed bed rest, there were so many obstacles. Plus, if we were lucky enough to have this baby I would need at least six weeks' recovery time before I would be allowed to have intercourse. I know he felt like my body was no longer available to him. In fact, in my current condition we couldn't be intimate in any way, because if my body was aroused it would only bring on additional contractions, and perhaps the complete onset of labor. We were told to be very careful in this regard.

One might be thinking that this seems like a pretty cool time to catch up on reading, or TV/laptop computer time, or phone time with friends, but I would argue quite the opposite, because I could do none of the above. Here's why: *All* of them gave me worse contractions, or I couldn't enjoy them due to the side effects of the medication. The terbutaline made my hands too shaky to hold a book. My effort to use our laptop computer became a nearly impossible task. I couldn't really use it flat on my back, and when I tried, it gave me contractions. In 2003, the iPad wasn't around yet, and even if it had been, I'm not sure it would have mattered. Simply talking on the phone was a curse. For whatever reason, my contractions worsened every time I had a conversation. Even my attempt to watch TV was disappointing. With limited channels available in the hospital, the morning and evening news (which would repeat over and over again) became boring for me. I reserved the twenty minutes of sitting-up time for eating my meals. Those precious minutes became crucial to me, because I was worried about getting bad acid reflux or indigestion from lying flat all day. Twenty minutes spread over three meals isn't a generous allotment.

I decided it was best to listen to my body and respect what it was telling me. After all, this was going to be for a limited time. If I did this right for just a few months, the reward in the end would be a great one, the best: the ultimate gift of a baby. I put my mind to it and became *very* comfortable with silence. I lay in that hospital room for hours with just the sounds of the machines around me. I got used to being alone in the relative quiet. In that time together with our baby I would rarely speak out loud to him, for that would break the silence I had become accustomed to. Once in a while I would sing softly or hum to him. Although I have a terrible singing voice, I wanted him to have a source of comfort in all the chaos he might be experiencing. "Amazing Grace" was my hymn of choice. It seemed apropos to wish for grace within me and for our baby. I spent a lot of time praying to God that He grant us this healthy baby boy. I reminded God I would do anything to get him home safely.

I had so many sweet friends and family who came to visit me during this time. And for that I am so very grateful. At first people would ask whether there was anything they could do or bring, and I would politely tell them no. But as my weight began to drop (the hospital food was not my favorite), I realized it was in my best interest, and the baby's best interest, for visitors to bring me something to eat. At every opportunity I asked for food. At one point I had lost so much weight that the hospital nutritionist was sent in to have a special meeting with me. I was told to either gain weight or I would be put on IV sustenance. I asked her to give me a few days and let me gain it the old-fashioned way. Fortunately, she agreed, and between the meals my mother brought in and the extras my friends provided, I was able to pack it on, putting on a few pounds in only three short days. The nutritionist was pleased, and we averted the IV from then on out.

Kevin visited me as often as he could, and his customary arrival time was late in the evening, on his way home from work. He would squeeze his body next to mine, a pair of sardines in my single bed. We would snuggle quietly for a bit while I asked Kevin to tell me about his day. There wasn't much for me to share. If all went well in my day, having nothing to report was actually a good thing.

One of the kindest people during my period of bed rest

was Dr. Cohen. In the evenings after he made his rounds, or after he was finished with deliveries for the day, he would come in to spend some time with me. Frequently it was as late as ten thirty or eleven p.m. He would quietly take a seat at the end of my bed and just engage in a friendly chat for a while. Oftentimes Kevin was there during his visit, so it presented an opportunity for all three of us to congregate. I was so impressed with Dr. Cohen's willingness to visit me. After all, he surely would have preferred to be at home with his own family or getting some much-needed rest. Yet he made the time to check in with me. I sincerely appreciated his visits, and it just reaffirmed for me what a caring doctor he was. If only we all could be so lucky as to have that kind of quality health care.

About a week or so into my bed rest, Kevin called me early one evening with a serious tone in his voice.

"Stacey, we need to have a talk."

What could possibly be so important at a time like this? Is the premature delivery of our baby not enough? I turned to the left as a bigger contraction took control over my body.

He continued. "Your mother has moved *all* of the artwork in the house. Every painting is in a different spot. I know she thinks she's doing us a favor and making things look fresh. It may even look better, but she did it without asking, and I like the way our art was arranged."

Kevin grew up in a home where things didn't change very often. In contrast, I grew up in a home where my mother literally changed artwork, upholstered couch covers, and rotated bed linens with the seasons. It was refreshing to her.

The new art placement probably did look better. But that didn't matter. The problem was that she hadn't asked whether she could do it, and it was our home, not hers.

"Please let me handle this. I don't want to talk about it anymore," I said. These days our conversations were brief—I was afraid of more big contractions, which could be brought about by lengthy or stressful discussions. Kevin understood that.

Later that night, my mother came into the hospital room, cheery and bright as usual. She was unbelievable. She would take care of all the responsibilities in our home, which included checking the mail, caring for the dog, buying fresh groceries, doing the laundry, cleaning the house, and much more. Then she would come see me. Occasionally she squeezed in a little shopping, but she would always have things ready at home again for the next day. She often took the time to massage my bedridden and achy body, which was a luxury like no other.

Today was a little different. I began, "Mom, I need to talk to you about something, and I just need you to listen and respect what I have to say."

My tone was very serious, and I continued. "I understand you moved some artwork around in our house. It's not sitting so well with Kevin, and while I'm sure it looks better than before, I need you to put it back, please."

"Okay," she said simply. End of discussion.

It was that short and sweet. A rarity for us.

Fortunately she took it in stride, and she returned every piece to its original position. We have quite a bit of art, so this was no easy task, I'm sure. Crisis averted. Contractions still under control. Husband happy again. Phew.

Roughly two weeks into my bed rest at the hospital, I started to really miss our dog, Jewel. She was, after all, much like our child. She used to sleep in our bed, which she did less as my belly grew. I was worried about her kicking the baby in the middle of the night as she shifted about, so I had been nudging her off increasingly. She was a true member of the family, and our struggle to have children made our relationship with our dog closer...probably not so unusual. I took Jewel on long walks and gave her lots of attention, and she came with us to my parents' house when we went for weekend visits. We were not by any means obsessive about her, but she was included in family events as much as possible. She was a fairly large but very well-behaved dog. Every time I lost a pregnancy, I could come home to Jewel and find her wagging her tail to greet me. She would gently rest her head in my lap as if to say, *I'm sorry, Mom.*

One sunny afternoon the nurse told me that she wanted to take me outside in the wheelchair for some fresh air. It was such a beautiful day, and I had not been outside since the day I had been admitted, fourteen days before. It would consume the majority, if not all, of my twenty minutes of "sitting up" time for the entire day, but I craved the sunshine and agreed it was worth it, though I also thought about how I would have to lie down later for the rest of my meals. As we got closer to the double glass doors of the hospital, I squinted to see things better. It looked like our car was at the entrance. And was that Kevin standing next to it? I was confused until I saw seventy-five pounds of pure joy leap out of the car. Jewel shook with excitement from her nose to the tip of her tail, her floppy ears making a fan in the sunshine. In her usual fashion when she got excited, she pulled her jowls back, greeting me with a toothy smile. Oh, how I had missed her! Between the two of us, I'm not sure who was happier. I'm certain she was confused as to why she hadn't seen me in so long, and usually a car ride meant a visit to the vet or a trip to the grandparents' house, but this was neither. And what were all these funny smells? She had to be wondering where she was. I burst into tears. I just couldn't believe my eyes! I was so thrilled to see her, and delighted that Kevin had thought of it. He had never mentioned the idea, but he had clearly clued into the fact that I was missing home, and that included Jewel. He must have prearranged it with the nursing staff. It was a surreal reunion, and I was a little embarrassed by my emotional reaction. I blamed it on my raging pregnancy hormones. As the tears poured down, Jewel licked my face and pranced all around me. For about ten minutes I just sat and stroked her head and body and loved on her. Our time together went by at warp speed, and all too soon it was time for me to go resume my horizontal position. I gave Jewel a huge hug and told her I hoped I would be home soon. She focused on me with her big brown eyes and tilted her head to the side, listening intently. Man's best friend. They are truly a gift.

The staff on my unit was incredible, and I got to know

them well during the three weeks I was in the hospital. In addition to the nurses, I also had the perinatologists rotating through to check on me every day. They performed a fetal fibronectin (fFN) test a couple times during my stay. It was similar to getting a Pap smear. The test evaluated the presence of fetal fibronectin, a substance present during pregnancy that connects the amniotic sac to the inner wall of the uterus. While not a clear prognostic indicator, it gave my health-care providers a better sense of how likely it was that I would go into active labor within the next week. It was supposedly a better predictor than evaluating only the frequency of my uterine contractions or the dilation of my cervix. Each time, the result indicated that I was not likely to go into labor, which was encouraging, to say the least. When you are admitted on serious bed rest and are as severely effaced and dilated as I was, the hospital staff talks to you a lot about getting just one day farther along in your pregnancy. Because *every day* matters. So the initial goal was to get me from twenty-four weeks to twenty-seven weeks, one day at a time. Once I achieved that, we breathed a huge sigh of relief.

When I was twenty-seven weeks pregnant, Dr. Cohen and Dr. Ryan Miller (my primary perinatologist) agreed I could be released to my home, since I had no other children to care for. They also knew I would have the help of my mother. I was somewhat tentative about returning home. It was reassuring to have all those nurses and doctors looking after me day and night, knowing that if, God forbid, something went wrong, I was in the best environment possible to manage the emergency. The crew over at Northside Hospital fully deserves their outstanding reputation. The high-risk unit managed my case beautifully, and I felt I was in good hands at all times. The caregivers gave me the confidence to go home and handle the contractions on my own. I had grown to understand my body well. I could sense when a contraction was going to remain minor and create less concern for the health of the baby. I could also detect when a small contraction would turn into a bigger, more serious contraction, giving us concern for further cervical dilation, not to mention the discomfort associated with it. During those, I needed to mentally transition into a temporary meditative state.

With a mix of nervousness and relief, I returned home. It was a welcome dose of nirvana. No more cumbersome monitors wrapped around my belly twenty-four/seven, no loud noises to wake me throughout the night, no poking and prodding to check me (except for the occasional doctor's visit). My routine at home began, as I religiously stuck to my bedrest orders as strictly as I had in the hospital. I slept in my own bed on our second floor at night, but would come down the stairs to our main floor for the duration of the day. My mother would kindly fix my breakfast, lunch, and dinner, which I consumed on the couch, where I lay horizontal all day long. Once in a while I would get up to go to the bathroom, and since it was summertime in Georgia, I would sometimes relocate to the couch on our screened-in porch until my next bathroom visit. The ceiling fans kept me cool enough, and the fresh air felt so good after my three-week hospital stay.

Jewel would lie down beside me and take an afternoon nap. She was clearly glad to have me home, but confused by my lack of attention and inability to get up off the couch to play ball with her. In the first few days I returned home, Jewel would bring me a tennis ball, place it gently by my hand, and sit waiting for me to throw it. It was something she had done countless times before. When I wouldn't toss it, she would whimper softly and rest her sweet head gently right next to my face on the couch. She just couldn't understand why I wouldn't play catch. After a minute or two of waiting, she would try to lick my face or start to wag her tail as if to say, *C'mon, Mom, I know you want to play with me!* And indeed I did. But, of course, I couldn't. It broke my heart to see her eventually lie down and just give up. After a few days she learned I was no longer an available playmate, and we simply became resting buddies.

At the end of the day, I would make my way back up the stairs and off to bed again. The only variation in my schedule was a shower once every three days or so, which was quick and exhausting. Even though I craved the warmth of the water running over my aching muscles, my body was not accustomed to standing; drying my hair became an impossible task because of the contractions it produced. My mother relocated an upholstered bench to our bathroom. After the shower I would spend a few minutes stretched across it, letting my hair fall off one end while my mother patiently ran the blow-dryer back and forth. I had to be so careful.

About once a week, I would make a trip to a doctor's office. I would either visit Dr. Cohen for regular checkups, or Dr. Miller for a more thorough screening (measuring the baby, taking a closer look at the developing organs, measuring amniotic fluid, evaluating the placenta, checking the length of my cervix, and more). With Kevin on the road for most of my bed-rest journey, my mother would drive me to the appointments. She had a minivan, and in keeping with my bed-rest instructions, I tilted the seat back so I could be as close to horizontal as possible, while still buckling my seat belt. At Dr. Cohen's office, I was surprised that I failed my initial gestational diabetes screening. I considered myself to be a healthy young woman, and I had now been eating totally nutritious food for several weeks at home, since my mother was my chef. Stephanie, Dr. Cohen's nurse, was very kind, and put me in a room where I could lie flat on an exam table while they continued to evaluate me. Luckily the secondary screening test showed that I did not have gestational diabetes, but I was not pleased with the testing process. Hanging out so long at the doctor's office and waiting for the results combined with the syrupy orange drink they gave me just added to my contractions.

Toward the end of my pregnancy, my husband came up with a great idea. He thought my mother could use a break and that he would invite his own mother down from New York to help for a while. Admittedly, he was ready for time with his own mother at the helm. It didn't take much to convince her.

When he made the call, I actually heard him plead, "Mommy, I miss you!"

Intuitively, Kevin's mom knew exactly what he was asking for.

"Do you want me to come down?" she asked, eager to please her son.

"Yeah, I could really use your help."

I get along very nicely with Kevin's parents, so it was fine with me that he asked for her help. She arrived only a couple of days later.

Little did he know the idea would backfire. Soon enough we ended up with not one, but two mothers, ready and willing to assist with my bed-rest care. My mother saw it as an opportunity to spend time with Maria, my mother-in-law, and the two ladies had a grand old time together. So much fun, in fact, that on several occasions I had to ask them to leave the room. Their incessant chatter literally gave me contractions. I was, however, very well cared for, and to this day I remain indebted for the gifts my mother and mother-in-law gave us during this difficult time.

NINE

EAT YOUR HAT

As time went by, we were thankful for every day we gained for our little boy's growth. A baby's weight, race, and gender are all major factors in predicting successful birth rates. Specifically, larger African-American girls have been proven to have the best survival rates. Our child had none of those characteristics. When they released me from the hospital I knew the chances of the baby surviving at twenty-seven weeks' gestation were good (greater than ninety percent), but definitely not ideal. There were a number of issues regarding the baby's long-term health that would be concerning. Making it to thirty weeks boosted the baby's chances up to greater than ninety-five percent survival. Finally, at thirty-four weeks' gestation, the chances of his survival leaped up another three points, to ninety-eight percent. If I went into labor, while it wouldn't be the optimal time to deliver, the baby should be relatively healthy after some time in the NICU (neonatal intensive-care unit). Slowly the days turned into weeks, and I began to breathe a sigh of relief.

The one final issue we were having with this baby boy was that he was not growing well in utero. While he had always measured small, his growth toward the end was just not substantial enough. Because of my multiple miscarriages, I would likely have been considered a candidate for genetic testing via amniocentesis. This perhaps could have provided some clues as to whether or not his small size was related to any particular cause. But because of my history of recurrent pregnancy loss and the fact that I was already having contractions, the risk that the procedure could put me into preterm labor was simply too high.

Dr. Miller was concerned the baby had something referred to as IUGR (intrauterine growth restriction). A diagnosis of IUGR means the baby weighs less than ninety percent of other babies at the same gestational age. There are a variety of underlying causes leading to IUGR, but in our case there was no indication of why our baby had it. The doctors increased the number of my perinatology visits to better evaluate the amount of amniotic fluid around the baby. They also monitored his growth, movements, and blood flow every few days. These measurements would determine whether it was better to keep prolonging the pregnancy or admit me for an early delivery.

To complicate things further, the baby was in a "frank breech" position, which means he was not only coming out bottom first, but his legs were in a pike position, with his feet up by his ears (like a diver would have them). Dr. Miller, Kevin, and I had a serious discussion regarding an attempt to manually manipulate my belly and move the baby into position for vaginal delivery. The procedure to rotate the baby involved my getting an IV…just in case it put me into active labor. I asked Dr. Miller to show me an example of what the rotation would feel like. Dr. Miller put his hands on my abdomen and gently began maneuvering the baby. The contractions and discomfort created by this was too much. I quickly stopped him. All we wanted was a healthy baby. In light of our boy's small size, I wanted every chance to let him grow and gain additional lung maturity. Along with the concern for IUGR, that seemed to be the other big issue I heard my doctors talking about—healthy lungs. If the baby didn't have mature, developed lungs, it would mean he would need medication and time in the NICU. A vaginal delivery was the last thing that mattered to me. I easily opted to have a C-section.

So all five of us—Kevin, my mother, my mother-in-law, Jewel, and I—plugged away until we began to reach the sweet end of my bed-rest days. It was about this time that my dear next-door neighbor, along with some other good friends, was kind enough to host a baby shower for me. I'd never expected to have the joy of a baby shower. The pregnancy had been so complicated, and the health concerns were always so intense that I was almost afraid to enjoy any of the traditions that often accompany the later stages of pregnancy.

I was so touched by the generosity of everyone there; it was an emotional day for me. As I lay stretched out on the couch in keeping with my prescribed bed rest, I relished this special time to celebrate our oncoming baby. It was also nice because I had not been able to shop for any of the items I needed. The crib we purchased was based purely on the recommendation of a friend, and I just figured that other than the very basics that would be needed with the baby's arrival, everything else could wait. I would have fun picking out a few things after our baby was delivered safely. The shower gifts gave me the opportunity to feel an excitement I had never allowed myself to feel before...for fear that the pregnancy would come to an abrupt and unexpected end. That is the ending I was accustomed to. I prayed so hard that this pregnancy would be *the one* that gave us the child we longed for.

At thirty-seven weeks, Dr. Cohen took me off the terbutaline and told me I could move around more. I was thrilled! *Freedom at last!* I was ready to live life again, even if it was a little bit at a time. One of the first things I did was go to the neighborhood swimming pool. It was summer in Georgia, and the heat was getting to my large pregnant body, as it would anyone in my condition. My mother and I arrived at the pool in the late afternoon, when it was unlikely that children would be frolicking about. Walking just the short distance from the car to the entrance of the pool exhausted me. As I opened the gate I saw we had the facility to ourselves. I rested on a lounge for a moment and kicked off my flip-flops, letting a contraction pass. As soon as it was over, I made my way to the shallow end, grabbed the handrail, and began my descent into the water. My mother watched like a hawk as I gingerly moved down a single step, pausing, and then one more, like a chameleon making his way down a branch. The surrounding water felt so foreign to me at first. The idea of doing anything besides lying horizontal in my bed almost sent me into a panic, but it was balanced by the thrill of being allowed to get out and do something—anything!

I splashed water first on my belly, then over my shoulders, which sent chills down my spine. Submitting to the urge, I glided into the pool, feeling more buoyant than I had anticipated. The water enveloped me as I floated along. The contractions lessened for the first time in months. I couldn't believe how therapeutic this simple dip in the pool was. I carefully swam a few laps, parting the water with a breast-stroke. *If I could only have completed my nearly four months of bed rest right here in the pool,* I concluded, *this wouldn't have been so bad!* Only twenty minutes later I returned to the steps, cautious not to push myself or drain my body and bring on contractions that would surely lead to full-on labor. I held on to the handrail and struggled to lift my body, a lead weight, up and out of the water. The experience was invigorating, refreshing, and yet peaceful all at once. I returned the following day and repeated the exercise.

After forty-eight hours of my being off the meds, my contractions were coming on strong. It was the middle of the night, and I woke Kevin, anxious that I was going into labor. These contractions were coming at least every five minutes, which was not entirely odd for me, but this time they were all intense. In the past few months, it was customary for most of them to be mild, scattered with moderate to severe ones. I phoned the doctor on call and explained my circumstances. He quickly put me back on the terbutaline, with the goal of getting me to my scheduled C-section date of September 9, 2003, now just five days away.

Surprisingly, I made it. We arrived at the hospital early the morning of September 9. That day is also my sister-in-law's birthday. We were happy it was not the anniversary of 9/11. Kevin and I both preferred not to have our baby born on that day if we could avoid it.

My experience that morning in the hospital was surreal. I had dreamed of this moment for almost thirty-two years, with the past three and a half months moving in slow motion. It had taken us five long pregnancies to get to full term. All we had to do now was get the baby out safely. I was not going to rest easily until I heard a loud cry from our son. Dr. Cohen was our doctor that day, which gave me great comfort. It was fitting: He had been on this long and difficult journey with us, and I felt as though he deserved to share in the joy if indeed today brought a happy ending. As a doctor who loves to deliver babies, he would do everything in his power, I knew, to make sure the delivery went as smoothly as possible. Darlene and Stephanie, two nurses in his office whom I knew well, were also scrubbed in and there to help. Their presence was a delight too, and we would all be able to rejoice in the delivery of this long-awaited child.

I was strapped down to the table, arms out in typical C-section fashion. My position reminded me of Jesus on the cross, and trust me, I was praying to Him and His Father at the time. Kevin was allowed in the room, and he readied our video camera to record the birth. Dr. Cohen talked us through each step as he began to free our precious miracle from my womb.

He interjected humor as he went along. "We were contemplating doing a gastric bypass while we were down here." And then he was serious again for a moment: "You'll feel lots of pressure."

Emerging from me was this child of God whom I'd been told would never make it. Kevin was filming over the sheet that prevented me from seeing what was happening.

"You doing okay?" he asked me several times.

"Yep. Getting a baby," I said, choking back the tears.

"Okay, Stacey, here comes lots of pressure." And Dr. Cohen pulled our son fully out of my body.

I knew the baby had been delivered, yet there was still silence in the room. *Why isn't he screaming yet? Isn't that what healthy new babies do?!*

As if reading my mind, Dr. Cohen lightened the moment. "Check out the size of that…foot!" he teased. "You have a son! Happy birthday to you," he broke out in song. "Thank God he looks like his mother!"

"He has lots of hair," added Darlene.

"Look what you got!" Dr. Cohen held our boy high above the curtain so I could see. "Hi, Mom," he spoke on behalf of our child.

A nurse took our baby from Dr. Cohen and placed him on a nearby table. As he carried the baby away Dr. Cohen called out triumphantly, "We did it!"

"Congratulations!" Stephanie and Darlene echoed his sentiments.

I wondered whether our little guy was okay. I still hadn't heard him cry yet. Kevin was peeking over the sheet, focused on holding the camera steady while he aimed a few yards away.

The nurse could tell he was straining to see what they were doing with the baby. "Come on over here, Dad." He beckoned Kevin to come closer. Left alone on the operating table, I held my breath while Kevin went to check on the baby. It gave me peace to know my husband was watching over our child; he has spent plenty of time in operating rooms. I knew he had the sense to pick up on whether anything was going wrong. Finally the baby screamed out. And he kept screaming. It got louder and stronger. There was no sweeter sound.

"All this crying is good for him," the nurse told Kevin. "Ten toes, ten fingers, all his little boy parts, a couple of ears. Y'all did a great job!" he said reassuringly.

Kevin filmed as they cleaned him, weighed him, measured him. He weighed in at five pounds, fourteen ounces. The baby had a bruise on his forehead, and they guessed that it came from his head rubbing up against my ribs for so long. They took a good look at his hips due to his frank-breech position. We were informed that he would need further evaluation to confirm that he did not have dislocated hips.

"Well, we know his plumbing works!" Dr. Cohen announced as our baby sprayed pee around the room. Everyone chuckled.

"He's so much bigger than I expected," Kevin kept

saying. This gave me some additional relief, especially after all the concerns about his size in utero.

"He's adorable, Stacey," Stephanie said with love in her voice.

"I'm trying to figure out who he looks like," Kevin said from afar. He looked over at me. "He's got your nose."

They wrapped up the baby and brought him over to me. Carefully placing the bundle next to my face, I now had a free hand to stroke his body. I turned my head to the side and kissed his cheek, then whispered into his ear, "I love you, babe." I kissed him again and again.

"I think she likes him," Dr. Cohen said endearingly as he looked over at Kevin.

It was a dream come true. For some people it's easy to have a child, which does not mean that you love your child less than we loved ours. But I do believe that when there is such a phenomenal struggle to have a child—something so easy for some and such a challenge for others—there is a different sort of appreciation in that moment for those of us who forged the onerous path. I took nothing for granted.

They completed the C-section and closed the incision. I thought about my new status as a mother. *If there is a reason to believe in God, this is it.* There are so many things that can go wrong when creating a human. Cells have to divide and form into all the right parts and function in all the right ways. There are countless opportunities for something to deviate from the proper path, and yet most of the time everything fits together the way it is supposed to. Now, that is something to marvel at.

And then, on top of that, my body had to perform as the carrier for the baby. I was becoming a believer again.

My surgery was complete and they brought the baby back to me. Kevin and I stared at the phenomenon before us. Our first angel on earth. One we got to keep for a while.

Thank you, God. Thank you for giving us the joy of this one. I promise I will do everything I can to take good care of him. To comfort him and raise him well. To always love him and be there for him. I will not let you, or him, down.

As they wheeled me out with Baby Boy Urrutia in my arms, our family greeted us in the hallway. They were already moved to tears at the anticipation of a healthy grandchild delivered. Later, my father told me that the smile, relief, and exultation on my face were visible from a mile away. It was an expression unlike any he had ever seen on me before.

We named our precious baby boy Tyler Cole Urrutia. Losing fourteen ounces, he weighed a mere five pounds when we brought him home. We followed up with a specialist regarding his hips, and the X-ray indicated that all was well.

He was not a particularly good eater, as it would take him nearly an hour to nurse (he didn't latch on well). My milk did not fully come in until at least a week after he was born. So for each feeding, he needed to be nursed and then supplemented with a bottle, which meant that with only an hour and a half between feedings, I was getting little to no sleep.

Tyler also had fairly bad reflux, so every time he ate he

was uncomfortable. He would fuss and pull his legs into his chest in discomfort while crying and spitting up. In an effort to make him feel better, we put him to sleep in the infant carrier or tilted him upright in his crib as often as we could. Truthfully, not much seemed to help; I think his body just needed a little more maturing time. I had waited so long for him already; what were a few more months of being patient? According to the doctors, the symptoms of reflux would eventually improve, and hopefully he would outgrow it altogether. For months Tyler had a witching hour that lasted from about six p.m. to eleven p.m. every night, when he cried almost nonstop. It was classic reflux or colic or whatever you read about in all the books that describe how anything and everything you do to try to make the baby stop crying simply doesn't work. It's true. I learned not to fight it. Our pediatrician encouraged me to let Tyler cry it out, so long as he wasn't hungry, hurt, sick, or needing a diaper change. Walking away or disregarding (to a certain extent) your baby is hard to do. I would wander into another room where I couldn't hear him, or fold laundry while the machines were running just to get a break from it for a little while. Between the lack of sleep and the incessant crying, the first few months were not easy. I had great help from family, which was a lifesaver, given how much Kevin was on the road with his job. Even though we had some hurdles to overcome, I was just so blissfully happy to have Tyler that nothing else mattered.

I fell into the routine of motherhood easily. Undeterred by total sleep deprivation, I absolutely loved it. Kevin was a more hesitant first-time father, somewhat timid because of how fragile Tyler seemed, given his petite size. Once I reminded him that babies wouldn't break and were "built to last," Kevin became more hands-on. One of our favorite things was to hold Tyler and watch him while he slept. We were mesmerized by his angelic face. And as we stared at him, we would sometimes whisper about how we could've made a mistaken decision based on statistics and not be holding our darling baby. By letting nature take its course, with all the uncertainty that involved, we had been blessed with this child.

Kevin had a rigorous schedule. After days of being on the road, he would come home from work and want to go pick Tyler up from the crib.

"Please don't wake him! If you do, he's all yours!" I would say. But Kevin couldn't contain himself, and beelined for the crib. My plea was a complete joke for two reasons: first, of course he would wake the baby, and second, I would be the one dealing with the consequences, because Kevin never got Tyler back to sleep in those days. I would need to nurse him or soothe him to get him back down again. That was just how it worked in our house while his reflux was so bad.

Tyler was a quickly socialized baby. We lived in a community where there were houses containing two, three, or even four children in each home, and everyone was just steps away. All the kids could walk to the public elementary school located at the entrance of the neighborhood. On a sunny afternoon, our streets were somewhat akin to a scene from a movie where the children run freely and happily home, with wide grins on their faces and joy in their voices. Except it was real. It was a great community, and we were lucky to live in a place where we were surrounded by such lovely people. When we arrived home from the hospital, the word spread, and everyone came to our house to meet our little man. I guess it's good that I was not overly concerned about germs. It's as though the entire community had been waiting for him, praying for his safe arrival. Unless a visitor was sick, I wasn't about to deny a visit.

We also had the most wonderful and generous Helping Hands group in our neighborhood. A letter came in the mailbox, notifying us of what we could expect: An organized group of volunteer neighbors would bring meals three times a week and a breakfast basket on Saturday mornings. These gifts kept coming for two months! I soon learned Helping Hands did this for anyone who needed some tender loving care. It could be for a family with a newborn baby like ours, or for someone who was battling cancer, or dealing with any other issue that required extra assistance. It was one of those things I was so truly grateful for that I couldn't wait to return the favor. Kevin's reaction to the help was quite comical. Having been raised in New York City, he was shocked by the notion of people reaching out to assist us in this way. It was a great blend of suburbia and Southern hospitality at its finest.

One very special outing Kevin and I made with Tyler in his first week of life was a trip to Dr. Goldsmith's office. Not only did we take the time to introduce our firstborn son to this fabulous doctor who had played such a key role in helping us bring Tyler into the world, but we also brought him a gift.

Upon arrival, the secretary escorted us to Dr. Goldsmith's office and asked us to wait while he finished seeing some patients. I was cognizant of other patients in the waiting room, who may have seen us walk in with a baby. I remembered how difficult it was to be at work surrounded by pregnant women, stories and photos of their newborn babies a regular part of our meetings. Perhaps seeing us with a baby in this setting gave the other patients hope that they, too, would one day be able to introduce their infant to their doctor.

While Tyler slept peacefully in his carrier, I placed an ornate hatbox on his desk. Dr. Goldsmith finally walked in, and instantly saw the item placed before him.

"What's this?" he asked, confused.

"Remember what you told us you would do if we had this baby?" I asked with a smirk on my face. He began to remove the lid to the hatbox.

"You told us you'd eat your hat," Kevin said with a smile. In the box were some utensils, a golf cap, and a Corona.

"I threw in the beer to make it go down a little smoother," I said.

He was clearly touched. "You know, nothing makes me happier than to have an outcome like this. Thank you so much for bringing this in!"

We visited Dr. Cohen's and Dr. Miller's offices, too. We made the rounds of all the people who had helped secure this little guy's life.

Subsequently, our lives finally became a little bit "normal" in the sense that we were typical parents of a baby whom we took absolutely everywhere. We traveled to New York, New Jersey, California, Hawaii, Florida, South Carolina, Virginia, and more in his first eighteen months. And we stopped focusing on trying to have a baby for a while, which was a relief. We inhaled life with our child, one deep breath at a time.

Not too long after Tyler was born, I ended up making the decision to become a stay-at-home mom instead of returning to work. It was a difficult choice, but it was the right one. During the first three months of bed rest, my position at work was secured by the Family and Medical Leave Act (FMLA). The FMLA requires that your employer allow twelve weeks of job-protected, unpaid leave for special circumstances. But even more valuable than that, I had a boss who was willing to hold my job for the remainder of my bed rest as well as the customary maternity leave. My departure from the company that past June was completely unexpected. I'm sure it hadn't been easy to have me at work one moment and gone the next, without even a transitional meeting to review urgent matters. When Dr. Cohen ordered me to the hospital to begin bed rest on that frightful day, I never imagined it would be almost four months later before I was allowed to move around in any way.

My predicament was this: If I returned to work, I would resume a busy and somewhat unpredictable travel schedule. In my case in particular, I had a husband who was always on the road for business. We would need a full-time nanny in order to cover us during the day and for overnight business. I couldn't figure out how to do my job well and meet Tyler's needs at home, besides the fact that I would be missing out on a tremendous portion of his childhood. While it was a strange adjustment at first, the transition to become a stay-at-home mother began to feel natural rather quickly.

TEN

A WOMAN OBSESSED

When Tyler was barely over a year old, I spoke to Kevin about trying to have another baby. I had always felt very strongly about having a family with more than one child. I grew up with an older brother whom I was close to, and wanted that same experience for Tyler. I also wanted him to have someone to share things with as Kevin and I aged. A brother or sister would give him someone to make decisions with down the road if need be, and it would give him the opportunity for a bigger family. I lacked multiple cousins and wanted that larger sense of family for myself and for my children.

Kevin was convinced. I stopped nursing Tyler at fourteen months, and we began trying to get pregnant again. We knew it could take a while to conceive, as it had previously. I secretly hoped my body would remember how to get pregnant and it would take only a few easy months.

After nine months of trying, we made an appointment with Dr. Goldsmith. My menstrual cycle had gone from a very predictable twenty-eight days to being all over the map. As I had experienced before, some months I had a twenty-four-day cycle, and other months I had a thirty-two-day cycle. My optimum ovulation time was a complete guessing game, and had it not been for those amazing ovulation-predictor kits, I would have been totally in the dark. My ideal days to make a baby were a moving target. Months earlier, Dr. Cohen performed a sonohysterogram to assure us that my uterus was clear. Nothing remarkable was found, so we were able to rule out any uterine adhesions, masses, or abnormal structures as a cause of my infertility.

Situated in the corner of Dr. Goldsmith's office was the hatbox we had given him less than two short years ago. He noticed us glancing at it.

"You know, I get a lot of special gifts from my patients, and I really don't have room to keep them all here in my office. However, your hatbox serves as a reminder for me and for my future patients that although I might have to share bad news with them, there's always a chance I may have to eat my hat. In cases like yours, nothing could make me happier."

"That's really great," was all I could muster. Just thinking about it brought tears to my eyes. I felt that if our story could give hope to even one single family, that was an accomplishment.

We explained to him that we had been struggling to get pregnant. It had been nine grueling months, and even the use of ovulation-detector kits had failed to help us conceive. I was getting frustrated. I felt it had been long enough, and my stress level surely wasn't helping us. Plus, with my complicated history and mysterious menstrual cycle, perhaps it was time to consider some other options. His game plan was to run some basic tests on Kevin first, as those were simpler and less expensive, and then we would move to evaluating me. My tests would commence in about a month, after the start of a new cycle.

Another month or more wasted. As usual I was impatient. I had to wait for my current cycle to end and a new cycle to begin so we could spend a month running tests. Then we would meet again to evaluate how everything looked before we would proceed. This was best, and I knew that, but it wasn't what I wanted to hear.

That month we had sex without a cause, appreciative of the respite from the procreative demands usually put on our sex life. Later that month I took Tyler out for some fun at a local playground. We were starved after a few hours of hardcore hide-and-seek. Rather than rushing home, I decided to treat us to lunch a local restaurant. The burger I ordered was stacked with cheese, grilled onions, lettuce and tomato, ketchup, and mayonnaise, just the way I liked it. My weakness was French fries, and I had an enormous pile of them on my plate. Famished, I took a huge bite of the burger. I nearly gagged. *That was so bizarre.* I thought about it for a moment. *The only time I get nauseous like this is when I'm pregnant. There's no way I'm pregnant. Wait. Maybe I am pregnant. It is possible. I have to go take a test and figure this out,* now!

I hurried Tyler along to finish his meal. The rest of my

food was dumped in the trash. Next to the restaurant was a drugstore. With Tyler holding my hand, I grabbed a test pack, paid for it, and headed to the restrooms. The only thing available was a family bathroom, so Tyler came in with me. Unsure of what to tell my son should he ask what I was doing, I told him to face the wall and play a guessing game with me. I squatted over the seat and peed on the test stick, then watched the urine make its way up and into the result area. I said the words aloud.

"Unbelievably positive."

"What's up, Mommy?" Tyler whipped around to see what had caught my attention.

My jaw hung open; I was shocked by what I'd just witnessed.

"Oh, I just learned something that took me by surprise. Everything's okay. In fact, everything is really good." To my astonishment the pale pink pregnancy line had appeared.

I couldn't wait to tell Kevin and decided to inform him in a creative way. We had stationery that had cartoon sketches of a man, woman, child, and dog on the front, representing, of course, Kevin, me, Tyler, and Jewel. Next to Jewel I scribbled a stick-figure baby as best I could, and on the inside of the card wrote the words, "Good news! We're pregnant!" It was my attempt at being cute, something I had not had the luxury of being before. We had been so tense around all of our pregnancies. This time I just felt it was all going to go well. Kevin was excited by the news. He reminded me that he had often felt my stress level accentuated the difficulties we had when trying to conceive. It was one of those "I told you so" moments. While he may have been correct in encouraging me not to feel such anxiety about our infertility, as a female living that reality, it was hard to simply turn off that switch in my brain. Nevertheless, we celebrated our good fortune, and I scheduled an appointment with Dr. Cohen.

A few days and several more positive pregnancy tests later, I called Dr. Goldsmith.

"Uh, guess what? You know those tests we planned on doing soon? We can put them on hold for now. Seems nature had a way of making things work on their own this month. Sometimes when you're not trying is when things work the best!" I informed him.

He was genuinely pleased.

It was a nice relief financially too. Not that we were unwilling to do what it took to have our next baby, but nature's way sure was a lot cheaper than via the infertility office! It's one of the things people going through infertility issues don't talk much about, because it's such a private subject. The financial aspect involved in overcoming infertility adds to the already stressful disposition in a household struggling with it on any level. People tend to be reserved about sharing details of either the cost of fertility treatments or the affiliated financial strain, even with the closest of friends and family.

As I began to relax a little bit, knowing that we were once again pregnant, I reflected on our lives since trying to start a family. There had been times in our baby-making days (or years) that were very taxing on Kevin and me, and we struggled through it for a while. It was a true test of the strength of our marriage, and I can understand how some couples don't survive it. The way I processed and managed the desire to have a family was entirely different from Kevin, and we didn't always agree on how to handle things. We would lose a pregnancy and I would want to start trying right away again, while Kevin would want a break. I would push to make sure we could have sex on exactly the right days to maximize our chances of conceiving, and Kevin wanted to be more carefree. That didn't fly with me, because he still traveled so much for his career. We had to "work" at being together. We both had been through the emotional loss of our babies. But it seemed to me that if I was the one physically going through all the losses, why did it matter to him if I was ready to start so quickly again? I was the one getting nauseous and going through all the surgeries and bleeding, etc. If I was willing to try again, shouldn't he be? We began bickering over little things that hadn't mattered before, because it all circled back to the bigger picture of us (especially me) wanting to have a family—and the constant failure we met with. Kevin now admits that many times he was ready to stop trying, but continued for my sake.

It was our (albeit not perfect) communication with each other, and our persistence and dedication to getting through it as a couple, that allowed us to weather many tough years. This season of our lives, when we struggled to complete our family, required tremendous patience.

While it would be ideal to say that when one of us was feeling down, the other was there to provide comfort, that really wasn't the entire truth. There were plenty of occasions when grief overpowered our ability to provide comfort to the other person. In fact, sometimes, my husband and I were not always in agreement on where we were headed next in our fertility journey. It was these times in particular that we needed to focus on the vows we had made to each other the day we married. It was a test of our decision to stay together.

Any marriage requires work and compromise, but our issues with infertility required a whole different level of commitment. In all honesty, we should have turned more to our faith as a means of helping us, but both of us were struggling with that. I felt anger and bitterness toward God and wondered whether there even was a God, and if so, why would He be bringing this upon us? Fortunately, our love for each other prevailed. That love allowed me to accept that my husband and I didn't have to share the same perspective. Instead, I needed to simply respect how he felt and honor that it was different, but not less important than the way I felt.

If we had not persevered through it as a team we would not have made it. That usually meant that one of us would give in to the other person based on who cared more about the subject at hand. With regard to pregnancy, I admit to being more stubborn, unrelenting in my wishes. In other (nonprocreative) aspects of our life, I gave in to Kevin's desires. We struck a balance, and ultimately our marriage survived.

I know there are many couples who can relate to this aspect of infertility and the additional strain it puts on a marriage. In a recent conversation with a friend regarding her infertility story, I learned she and her husband were attempting to have a second child, but were struggling to conceive and carry another. On average, it took them close to a year to conceive between pregnancies, and they experienced numerous ectopic pregnancies, where the embryo implants somewhere other than the uterus, such as the fallopian tubes. One of the ectopic losses was so dangerous that my friend nearly lost her life.

As I talked with her, we related on so many levels, as if we were members of a secret club, one requiring special entry. And let me be honest: I'm not proud to be a member. We discussed how it was very hard for our friends who have not dealt with infertility issues to understand what we were going or had gone through. While bystanders might try to say the right things, most people fumbled over their words. It was done innocently and without malicious intent. They meant well, but so often their words were hurtful. She pointed out that frequently people would say to her that she "had it easy" with only one child. They were not consciously considering that she might be trying to have another and just hadn't been able to do so.

The other thing we talked about was how hard it was to be going through infertility and not be able to share the struggle with anyone. She said she regularly felt as if someone would ask how her day was and she couldn't give an honest answer. Her thoughts were consumed by the desire to have another child, yet she couldn't openly discuss it. There were the private medical issues. There was the consideration of adoption. And to top it off, there were financial issues that made it practically impossible for them to consider seeking assistance from a reproductive endocrinologist. It was all so awkward. As a result, she had just pulled away and backed off from social outings to get herself in a "better place."

After a good amount of self-reflection while she was more socially withdrawn, she told me she felt spiritually happier and physically healthier than she had in a while. Despite her and her husband's disappointments, their marriage was good. If things continued to go well for the next couple of years, they might be in a better financial position that would open up some options. In the meantime, she sensed that people wondered why she seemed distant.

The thing is, this whole infertility thing doesn't just go away overnight, in a few months, or even in a few years. She and her husband have had to figure out how to get to a peaceful place with it. I hope that those of you reading this who have not been through any infertility difficulties can try to understand that people like us are just trying to figure out how to handle it; it may take us a while, sometimes years, to resolve it. And for us, it may not result in the child or children we hoped for. That can be devastating, which is why it is so important to find solace despite the outcome. We must learn to see the adversity as a gift, the purpose of which we may have not yet figured out.

I told my friend that some of the best advice given to me was by a dear friend who spent more than ten years and a hundred thousand dollars trying to have a baby. After we had Tyler and were trying to get pregnant again, she simply explained to me that I should "pray for peace."

"By praying for peace," she explained, "you accomplish a sense of peace in your life regardless of how you get there, and regardless of the outcome to your problem. You learn to find comfort in living in the moment, and with that, gratitude for the other blessings you have been given."

I desperately needed to listen to her words. I was obsessed with the minutiae of my menstrual cycle. The first half of the month I was bleeding and waiting to ovulate. The middle of the month I spent detecting the day I would ovulate and consequently timing intercourse with my husband (and figuring Kevin's travel schedule so he would be at home at the ideal time). The latter part of the month I waited for the days to pass until I could take a pregnancy test to find out whether we had been successful. I never waited to bleed. I used a pregnancy test early every month, and then felt disappointed if it was negative. Then I spent days bleeding and moping. And the next month it would start all over again. That was my cycle. It wasn't a healthy way to live. The mental and emotional tension it put on my body was not conducive to promoting conception! And yet I bet most women with infertility issues behave in a manner similar to mine. They become consumed with it.

At the time, praying for peace sounded like a good suggestion. Since then I have resorted to her advice for all types of challenging situations our family has endured. I try to believe God will handle the means to get there if we do our best and pray for peace.

ELEVEN

PLANNING FOR PINK

Our sixth pregnancy was confirmed, and harmony returned to our lives. I was monitored closely from then on by both Drs. Cohen and Miller. This time my hCG numbers were soaring. At approximately twelve weeks' gestation, we opted for a nuchal translucency test with this pregnancy as well, and the results indicated there was no concern about the chromosomal or congenital heart defects the test could predict. I was nauseous as could be and happy to be feeling that way. In fact, it was the sickest and most exhausted I had ever felt, and I welcomed every moment of it. I figured it meant I was still pregnant; so as long as I felt cruddy, I was still carrying a baby. My exhaustion was due in part to chasing a younger one around. Tyler was one active little fella, not uncommon for a boy of his age. He was a petite but capable two-year-old.

His verbal skills were through the roof. We often tell

our friends a story of how Kevin came home very late from one of his business trips when Tyler was only fifteen months old. Kevin had not seen either one of us in nearly a week. Tyler was already in bed, sleeping soundly. Later that night while we were asleep, Tyler began to cry and call out for us. We both woke up, startled. It was uncommon for him to awaken in the middle of the night. I could tell Kevin was eager to go in and console him.

I looked at Kevin and said firmly, "Don't go in there. He'll settle down soon, I bet, and put himself back to sleep."

"Stacey, I haven't seen him all week. I wanted to go in there when I got home, and now that he's awake it's killing me. I really want to go in and comfort him."

I gave him a look that was clear: "Here's the deal. If you go in there, he's all yours for the rest of the night."

"I'm going in!" And Kevin rushed out of the room. I turned up the video monitor to watch and listen in for a moment. I could see Kevin walk into Tyler's bedroom.

"Tyler, buddy, what's the matter?" Kevin asked him in a soft voice, not truly expecting a response.

Tyler was standing in the crib, holding on to the rail like an angry little man. Kevin leaned in and gave him a gentle kiss on each cheek.

Sure enough, when Tyler realized he had an audience, he abruptly said, "Daddy, Ty-Ty night-night all done." Tyler stared at him with a frustrated look on his face. Kevin was shocked that he'd spit out a full sentence. Kevin had been gone only five days.

Kevin composed himself and tried talking sense into

him. "No, Tyler, you have to go back to sleep. It's the middle of the night and everybody is sleeping."

Tyler held firm and looked at him sternly. He pointed to the ceiling and said, "No, Daddy, light's on!"

Kevin was baffled by the full conversation they were having. In that short week, Tyler had begun to speak in simple sentences. Kevin picked up his son and carried him downstairs. As I heard him prepare a bottle, I drifted back to sleep. I later discovered that Kevin fed him while they watched some late-night TV together. Not exactly great parenting, but at least he was taking care of him rather than handing Tyler off to me. Apparently it took Tyler a good hour or two to fall asleep in Kevin's arms. Kevin carried him back up the stairs and gently laid our angel in the crib, then returned to bed exhausted but satisfied.

The next morning he told me it was one of those special moments in life with Tyler, and he didn't regret it one bit. While there is a logical approach to sleep training, he was glad he followed his heart and went in to spend some time with his child.

Another classic, memorable story with Tyler occurred when he was about twenty months old. I was preparing to bathe him, and as I reached down to help lift him in, he resisted.

"No, Mommy, all by myself," he said, pushing me back with his hand.

As he started to climb over the edge of the tub there was

a moment where he teetered with one leg in and one leg out. I could hear his crotch screeching against the porcelain. I looked at him with my face expressing concern for his discomfort.

He promptly and with complete reassurance said, "Don't worry, Mommy, my 'boys' are okay!"

Kevin had just arrived home from an out-of-town business trip with his luggage still in tow. I called out to him in a voice that was clearly a little perturbed. He was not getting his usual friendly greeting from me.

I began to lecture: "We need to have a talk. Our toddler just referred to his testicles as his 'boys.' If he brings that up in his Mother's Morning Out program, *you* will be the one explaining it to his teacher."

Kevin, rightfully so, defended himself.

"Well, I had to teach him to call them something, and I don't think we want him walking around in public talking loudly about his 'testicles' should he decide to bring it up, right?"

Point well made. I conceded and apologized to Kevin. To this day, if need be, we still call them the "boys," but in our own home we use all the correct names for all private body parts.

As to be expected, with Tyler's profuse ability to engage in conversation, there was lots of discussing this new baby growing in my belly. Tyler got to come along on the ultrasounds and see little baby Urrutia growing and developing.

My hCG levels were bumping up nicely, and my cervical length (a good indicator as to whether I would retain the pregnancy) was checked at least once every couple weeks by Dr. Miller. Both were looking better than ever.

With all the ultrasound monitoring, we figured out early this time that it was a baby girl. I was thrilled with this revelation! We would be having a boy and a girl in our house. It was what I had always imagined, because it was what I knew, growing up with a brother. And it meant I would get to experience raising both genders. Shopping trips to the mall that involved the color pink, mani-pedis together, braiding hair, father-daughter dances—those were just a few of the images that instantly flooded my mind. It was easy for me to envision our future family Christmas card with Mom, Dad, handsome Tyler, Jewel, and beautiful Baby Girl Urrutia.

Kevin, on the other hand, was totally apprehensive at the idea of raising a little girl. He had no idea how to handle one, and I think he could only envision all the boys in his little girl's life he would have to try to keep away. He is a natural protector, and just thinking about that level of responsibility made him quiver.

One of his favorite sayings was, "With a boy you only have to worry about one penis. With a girl, you have to worry about all of them."

The most special thing about this time in my life was that my best friend in the Atlanta area was also pregnant. Allison Carr was due only a couple of months ahead of me, so it was fun for us to be pregnant together. Her daughter, Madison, was the same age as Tyler, and they were the best of friends. When both our children were only about six months old, Allison and I had met in a local toddlers' music class. She was my source of sanity at that time, and I was hers. As I explained, Kevin was often out of town or late to return home. Likewise, she had a husband who worked late, so we regularly spent hours upon hours together, wrapping up the day with dinner in one of our homes and even bathing the kids at the conclusion of a playdate. Then we would send Madison or Tyler home in the other's pajamas. As a result, we became quick companions during what were some difficult and long, otherwise lonely days. Allison was and is like family to me. We were overjoyed with the idea that our second children would be so close in age.

When I found out we were having a girl we instantly began discussing names. We discussed girl and boy names for Baby Carr; Allison and her husband, Steve, were not finding out the gender of their baby (a bit tricky for them, as she is a pediatrician). After many lists were created, the one I liked the most for us was Tess, and it just seemed to stick. Kevin had vetoed many others, but this was one he was willing to consider. We decided to think about it for a while.

Christmas of 2005 came along, and it seemed like one of the most joyous times for us. Other than severe nausea, my pregnancy had been unremarkable. Tyler was the perfect little two-year-old toddler, making our holiday truly magical. He was so excited, and understood the spirit of Christmas for the first time. What a pleasure it was to have a child bring cheer into the house during the holiday season. We sang "Happy Birthday" to baby Jesus, and all three of us slept under the

Christmas tree, waiting for Santa to bring gifts and fill our stockings. I was about twenty weeks pregnant, and finally feeling better. Allison and I had just gone shopping together for some new maternity clothes. I felt good sporting some better-looking outfits than when I lay in bed during my bed-rest days with Tyler. I had the blessings of family around me, and a healthy child on the way. On Christmas morning, I can remember thinking about how happy I was.

Shortly after the holiday, I made a visit to my grand-parents' home in Hilton Head. With my car packed, I stopped by Dr. Miller's office to get clearance before heading out for the five-hour ride. He checked my cervix and the baby's vitals, as well as all the other basics to make sure things looked good. I received his approval, and he informed me that my cervix was the longest it had ever measured.

Tyler and I made our way on the road (Kevin was absent due to a business trip). My grandfather had not been well, and was unable to join us in Alpharetta for Christmas that year. I loved him dearly, and wasn't sure how much longer we would have him with us. I wanted to make sure we got to Hilton Head to see him, especially near the holidays. I played it safe and got out of the car to walk several times on the road trip. It was good for my circulation, and what the doctor had recommended I do. We made it to their home and I unloaded the heavy bags. Our visit was lovely and special. Tyler just adored his great-grandfather "Bopa" and great-grandmother "Nona." Without incident, we returned to Alpharetta only a few days later.

The next couple of days passed without anything

seeming noticeably different. The only substantial incident that I recall was when I got very frustrated changing Tyler's bedsheets. He had a heavy queen mattress, and we safeguarded him with rails on each side and one on the end. They were a brand that conveniently allowed you to make the bed without removing the rails, but for some reason they were not moving up and down easily. I must have spent thirty minutes struggling to get clean sheets on. I was hot and bothered, and it wasn't in a good way.

Shortly after making the bed, I remember having a few minor contractions, but nothing that seemed significant. They were little ones, and I had experienced them before with this pregnancy. They were considered acceptable by both Drs. Cohen and Miller. I went about my day, no concerns on my mind.

The next morning I woke up and was going through my normal routine. I had snuggled with Tyler for a while and we made the beds, had an early breakfast, and were just getting ready to play. We're both early risers, so it was only a little after seven a.m. Suddenly I felt like I had urinated in my pants. They were soaking wet. *I've heard of incontinence during or after pregnancy, but this is ridiculous!*

I quickly moved to the toilet and was shocked to see that the clear liquid running down my legs didn't look or smell like urine. I guessed it was amniotic fluid. I had read about water breaking when I was late in my pregnancy with Tyler, but had never experienced it due to my C-section. In an instant, I realized my water had broken, and my brain immediately went through the all-too-familiar process of realizing I was losing the baby.

This precious baby. How can this be? I'm twenty-two weeks pregnant. This isn't how it's supposed to go. Especially after all we've been through. We've had enough losses. This one was supposed to work, and it was going so well.

Tyler was calling for me from the other room. Kevin was out of town in Raleigh, North Carolina, preparing for an early case. I squeezed my legs as tightly as I could but continued to drip amniotic fluid. I was desperate for a solution to a problem that had no fix.

I called out, "Tyler, can you get the phone for Mommy, please? I need it quickly, honey! I'm sitting on the toilet, but I need you to bring me the phone."

I concentrated on sounding firm so he would react fast, but not so panicked that I would scare him. I went into automatic mode and focused on remaining calm. If nothing else, the one thing I had plenty of in this situation was practice.

God bless that little guy—he brought the phone to me right away. While still on the "throne," I promptly called Dr. Cohen's office, and he called me right back—the operator hadn't wasted any time reaching him. I explained the circumstances, and he asked me to drive to his office right away, which we both felt I could do. I was not having active labor pains, so it seemed reasonable, and it was the fastest way to get there during rush hour. He wanted to evaluate me without delay, and sending me to the hospital first would postpone the exam.

With Kevin unavailable, I hung up from Dr. Cohen and called Allison. I figured she was my best solution to both child care and transporting me to the hospital. Plus, she could keep me calm if I started to lose it. She was my rock when Kevin was absent. I reached her right away and told her what was happening. As a friend and a doctor, she would understand how serious this was. I knew that after Dr. Cohen's office, my next stop would be Northside Hospital. I didn't require an ob-gyn to tell me I was losing this baby. He would simply confirm it for me. The intellectual side of my brain had all the answers already. The emotional side of my brain was the one making me go through every step just to make sure some miracle wasn't going to save this baby, the same kind of miracle that gave us Tyler.

I made my plans with Allison and hung up the phone. The next call was tougher. I dialed Kevin. I predicted I would get his voice mail. *How do you leave a message for something like this? "Hi, sweetie. I called to tell you I'm losing the baby. I'm really sorry. When you get a chance, please come home." Does it go something like that? God, please let him pick up the phone, please....* Of course there was no answer. Keeping my emotions in check, I pretended (for Kevin's sake and for Tyler, who was listening in) to be strong. I left a message along those lines and prayed it sounded okay. It was all so heartbreaking. So crushing. I felt as if I were always calling him with devastating news. When would it end? Thank goodness we had Tyler. Numbed by the pain of my new reality, I tried to focus on the joy he brought us in an effort to keep myself on track and get through this. He still needed me, even now, during this crisis.

I made my way off the toilet and stuffed my pants with the thickest pad I could find in the house. Luckily I had saved a couple that were given to me after Tyler's birth. They were monster-sized, and should hold more than the usual amount of fluid. I quickly dressed, and as I continued to leak more fluid, I rushed us into the car, putting a towel on the seat to catch what my pad and pants wouldn't. I figured today would be an embarrassing day when it looked like I had peed in my pants. Normally I would have been horrified by that thought, but right now it was of little concern. The dark sweats I wore would help hide any wet spots, and the soft, comfy fleece would help me stay warm during the long day ahead. At twenty-two weeks' gestation, I didn't even look pregnant in this outfit.

It is here that I feel I begin to owe my best friends my greatest gratitude. And it starts with Allison and Steve. Without hesitation, they dropped everything and rushed to my rescue. I truly don't know what I would have done without friends like them, both physically and emotionally.

Steve stopped whatever he had planned at work that day. When we all met at Dr. Cohen's office, Allison stayed with me and Steve took the children. Since their daughter, Madison, and Tyler were best friends, for the kids this was an average day. Perhaps they sensed that something wasn't quite normal, but from their angle, the day just got better.

Allison told me later that Steve took them to a nearby McDonald's to waste some time while we figured out what would happen next. It had a great indoor playground for the kids, and he thought it would be a fun way to spend the morning. In an effort to distract Tyler from what had transpired at home (or maybe just to be a fun, cool dad), Steve gave them a special treat of milk shakes, which neither one of their little two-year-old bodies was accustomed to. Apparently they sucked the drinks down quickly...and out they came on the other end, simultaneously! Steve rushed both kids to the potty, as they had nearly spontaneous diarrhea from the milk shakes. Poor guy. Such a great idea, but, boy, did it backfire.

In the meantime, back in the exam room, Dr. Cohen evaluated me and spoke to Allison and me about the circumstances. He told me there was basically a total loss of amniotic fluid and I needed to be ready to deliver the baby. He was going to call Northside Hospital and make plans for my arrival there. We spoke about the condition of delivering a baby at twenty-two weeks and kept the conversation brief. It seemed fairly clear to me that babies born that early don't survive even in the best neonatal intensive care units, which Northside Hospital had. It would be up to Kevin and me to make the final decision as to whether or not we should attempt to save the baby.

While Dr. Cohen left the room, Allison and I got teary-eyed as we looked at each other and quietly talked about the options, or lack thereof. It was as though a death sentence had been given but the execution had not yet occurred. I knew I was the lifeline for this child, yet I could no longer continue to sufficiently provide life for our daughter. My body had failed again. Something had gone terribly wrong.

It's very difficult to describe the guilt, anger, and frustration that surged through me. As parents, it is our instinct to protect our children from harm. During late-pregnancy loss like this, when it was *my* body failing to safeguard our baby, it was perhaps what I would consider the ultimate self-disappointment. There was no one to blame but me. I realized there were lots of other women this happened to, and I was not alone in this predicament. Intellectually, I knew it was not my "fault" because I had done something wrong or been a bad person. Quite the contrary: I had been trying to do everything right.

I vaguely remembered a discussion that took place early in my pregnancy. Based on my high-risk status, Dr. Cohen suggested I receive a cervical cerclage (a surgical procedure in which the cervix is sewn closed to help an incompetent cervix, or cervix that dilates and effaces early, remain closed, thus preventing premature labor). In contrast, neither my repro-ductive endocrinologist nor my perinatologist recommended that I have one. After all, my cervix was measuring better than it had during any other pregnancy. There was uncertainty as to whether or not I had a truly incompetent cervix, which left it up for debate. The procedure was not without risk of miscar-riage, and we had been trying to reduce that risk. In the end, we opted to forgo the cerclage.

As I sat in bewilderment at my situation, I wondered whether that had been a horrible mistake. The reality was that it was too late to fix it, and who knows whether my body would have failed regardless. I believed every doctor involved in my care was trying his best to help me deliver a healthy baby, and hindsight is always 20/20. I shifted my attention back to the present calamity.

Steve returned with the kids, and we all got into one car to make the ride to Northside Hospital. I left my vehicle at Dr. Cohen's office, figuring we'd get it sometime later. I called my parents and they were on their way over to help. Devastated at the news, they had dropped everything as well, and knew it would be a long few days. They were always great with helping to take care of Tyler, and with Kevin being out of town, they could get to Atlanta fast to assist. I think they wanted to be there. It was, after all, going to be the birth and loss of a granddaughter for them, too.

When Allison and I walked into the Northside labor and delivery department, they looked at her to check in, not me. She was the more pregnant one, due a couple months ahead of me. It was January, and Allison was due in March. We gave each other a sarcastic look that said, *I know—isn't this a ridiculous scenario we shouldn't have to be in?*

My mouth was dry and it was hard to speak. "No, it's me you need to check in. I am only twenty-two weeks pregnant, but my water broke and I'm here to deliver the baby."

Steve arrived, and he and the kids joined us in the waiting area. Kevin finally called me and I spoke to him softly, since the children were present. I brought him up to speed on the analysis Dr. Cohen had given and told him I would talk to him again when we learned more from the doctors at the hospital. Kevin made plans to get back to Atlanta immediately. We didn't have a long and drawn-out conversation. I was worried about getting too emotional, and felt there wasn't much to consider. We would go through the motions of evaluating our options, but nature had made its decision for us, and things were spinning out of our control.

It was only a short wait before they put me on a stretcher and took me to see the perinatologist, who could evaluate how much amniotic fluid I had lost. As I expected, the news wasn't good. Even worse, not only had I lost most of it, but the tear was so large that as I was generating new fluid it was simply leaking out.

"Can I lie tilted back at an angle, so my body will hold the fluid while the tear heals? Or even somewhat upside down?" I pleaded.

Their advice was given in a sad but straightforward and simple tone: The tear was such that even with all the maneuvering in the world it was impossible for my body to heal the wound. I couldn't regenerate a sufficient amount of amniotic fluid to carry the baby long enough to deliver a healthy child. Even if I could make it for a short time, it was likely an infection, or some other problem (such as labor) would ensue.

With each bit of news that was reported to me, I got increasingly calm. Instead of becoming frantic and panic-stricken, I remained quiet and in complete control. It was almost as though I were no longer in my body, but rather looking down on it from above, feeling sorry for myself, watching it from afar. As if it were some other person's nightmare. Perhaps losing four other pregnancies had given me the ability to manage this trauma better than I would have expected. Surely I would have to process my emotions later. For now, anesthetized by the pain, I was surprisingly tranquil.

Ultimately, I knew we were having this baby soon. What concerned me most was Kevin getting back in time for her arrival. When our daughter came into this world, we would be faced with a choice: Did we ask the doctors to go through extreme measures to try to save a baby born at twenty-two weeks, or did we allow nature to take its course?

As they wheeled me back out of the perinatology room, my father arrived from Greensboro, Georgia, and relieved Allison and Steve so they could go home with the kids. My mother was tied up in an appointment, and while she planned to come that night, my father didn't wait for her. As a parent, I now better understand the saying that was shared with Kevin by a dear friend: "You are only as happy as your least happy child." I think as much pain as I was in, my parents felt my pain equally. They might not be struggling through the day-to-day journey of it, but their hearts ached for Kevin and me just thinking of what we were about to go through. I'm sure Kevin's parents felt the same.

They wheeled me back to my hospital room and we waited for Kevin and my mother to arrive.

In the meantime, I had a conversation with a dear friend of mine, who is a pediatric occupational therapist (OT). She and I grew up playing tennis together in South Carolina. Even though I lived in Hilton Head and she lived in Florence, South Carolina, we toured the Southeast together playing in tournaments, so our families were very close. After college, we reconnected when we discovered that we lived only a couple miles from each other in Alpharetta. She and her husband had their first son only a few weeks after Tyler was born. The boys were good toddler friends.

As a pediatric OT, she happened to be a feeding specialist who had spent time in the NICU of Northside Hospital and knew the details of working with preemies very well. She and her husband worked with autistic children and many other kids who needed any kind of occupational therapy, speech therapy, help with nutrition, etc.

I could count on her as my go-to girl for some honest answers. I knew she would give me the cold, hard truth. I asked her bluntly what her opinion was of attempting to save a baby born at twenty-two weeks. A tenderhearted woman who sees the best- and worst-case scenarios with prematurely born babies, her advice was as I expected: The complications from delivery and other postpartum factors would make it a very long road for this baby and for our family—if the baby even survived it, and that was unlikely.

Her comments matched those of the perinatologist, and all the nurses and doctors who rotated through my hospital room. We were told that the earliest babies surviving premature births were generally at twenty-four weeks' gestation, so the hope of our baby surviving at twenty-two weeks was a real stretch.

My mother arrived at some point between the blur and chaos of the information that was coming to us. My parents made plans with Allison for taking care of Tyler and Jewel for the remainder of the day. Kevin had not yet arrived, and they were hesitant to leave me alone at the hospital. I felt so bad for my mom and dad, too, losing another grandchild. It was sad for all of us. Mom greeted me with the *we're gonna make it through this too* look I'd seen many times before. My parents stand by their children through thick and thin. In good times and bad, they have always supported us. To say the least, I was grateful. They were there for me and Kevin, and they were there for Tyler, who adored his grandparents. He would need them while Kevin and I were absent both physically and, at times, emotionally for the next forty-eight hours.

Kevin's flight from North Carolina finally made it into the Atlanta airport, and he drove straight to the hospital. I was overcome with relief when he walked through the door. I felt as though I had been absorbing a lot of information and managing the crisis alone, and now he could be there to share it with me. It was so important to me to have him present for this, and that we go through this together. I had the sense our daughter wouldn't live long—assuming she survived the birth —but I didn't know for how long. I wanted us to be able to hold her, and for her to have a sense of being together with her parents, even if it was only for a few minutes.

As he walked into the hospital room he saw I was drowning in my sorrow. The control I had exhibited thus far finally cracked at my surface, and a flood of tears erupted from me. He later said the blood drained from my face, and my pale, grief-stricken exterior left my eyes hollow, devoid of the joy that only yesterday radiated through me. The shadow of death was creeping in on us. My demeanor confirmed his fears, and he realized in an instant that we were going to lose the baby for sure. Kevin explained to me that he thought, despite what I told him over the phone, that there would still be a way to save the baby. That the doctors would have figured *something* out. I watched as his body went limp with disappointment.

It was January 11, 2006, and we were about to make one of the toughest decisions of our lives. Kevin and I held hands and sat for a long time, staring at each other, unable to find the words of comfort we each longed for. We spoke quietly and I slowly regained control of my emotions. We focused on trying to make the right choice for the baby, for my body, and for our family. My parents knew this was a decision only Kevin and I could make. They left the hospital to manage things at home.

Shortly after Kevin arrived, Dr. Cohen came in and spoke with us. He stood at the foot of my hospital bed, compassion and pain exuding from him. There were not many words exchanged, but they were simple and direct. We knew Dr. Cohen well by now, and Kevin asked him to be honest.

"Tell me, Dr. Cohen, what would you do if this were your child?"

"I would suggest that you not go through extreme measures to save her. She would likely be a very, very unhealthy child, *if* she even survives. In my opinion it would be best to let nature take its course." He went on to explain, "Because of the size of the tear in your amniotic sac, we need to deliver the baby. If we wait to delay her delivery in an attempt to save her, it's probable that you would develop a very severe bacterial infection. That would present a serious risk to your health."

We valued every word he said. None of us took this decision lightly.

We had let nature take its course before.

TWELVE

THEN THERE WAS TESS

We decided it was best to start a medication that would bring on my labor and force me to deliver our baby girl. The plan, however, involved two steps: First, Dr. Cohen would insert a seaweed plug into my cervix to help it dilate. I was familiar with this, since it was used during the loss of our first baby, when I was almost eighteen weeks pregnant. Next we would begin the oxytocin intravenous drip the following day for the actual delivery. That meant waiting overnight for everything to begin.

As Kevin and I contemplated the fate of our baby, his phone rang. I heard bits and pieces of the call before Kevin stepped out of the room. Here is Kevin's recollection of that call:

My cell phone rang a short while after our discussion with Dr. Cohen. As I glanced at the caller ID, I remember Stacey looking at me as if to say, Do you really have to answer that? *Then it quickly turned into,* If you must, then make it quick. *She communicated in spousal sign language with nothing but the eyes.*

I answered the phone because it was a fellow coworker, and I knew he was aware of our current situation. Therefore he must have been calling for a very important reason. I also surmised that he was calling me from the annual Southern Association of Vascular Surgery meeting, or SAVS, which was a very important yearly conference, one that I had never missed.

As soon as I answered, he immediately apologized for calling me at this very difficult time, and quickly explained the reason for his call. He said that Dr. David Rosenthal had walked by the company's booth and was asking for me. When my colleague explained my absence, David insisted that he get me on the phone immediately. He then asked permission to pass the phone to David and I agreed.

The easiest way to explain David is that he is a larger-than-life sort of character. He is an extremely accomplished vascular surgeon, inventor, dedicated triathlete, mentor, husband, father, and now grandfather, just to name a few. But most of all, for me he had become a dear friend throughout the course of our work together. I had often confided in him over the years about our pregnancy losses, because he and his wife had also tried for many years before being blessed with three boys of their own. While our journeys were somewhat different, I knew he could really appreciate what I was going through, and his compassion and insight often gave me hope when I was feeling hopeless.

When I answered the phone, David started with, "Hey,

Kevy boy. I know you are going through a very difficult time right now...." Then he proceeded to tell me that he and his wife had been in the same situation, in that very same hospital, almost twenty-six years ago. They had experienced the tragic loss of a baby boy at just twenty-four weeks, and had chosen not to pursue extraordinary measures to save the baby. He spoke briefly about how gut-wrenching the experience had been for him, and how it was just "nature's way." But most of all, he wanted us to know that his heart went out to us and that he was thinking of us in this painful time. In that moment, I felt peace and gratitude for the kindness and compassion he had conveyed to me. He had done so in a way that only someone who had walked in my shoes could. I firmly believe that God speaks to us through others, and I am thankful that he sent David to me that day.

It was our last night together with our daughter. Every second with her counted. My body, the failing vessel for this life I so desperately wanted to save, and this little baby, joined for the last few hours of her life. It was agonizing for me to think of her fate. I tried to block my brain from processing her future and to focus on the here and now. What could I say to her? How could I console her? I was her earthly mother until she was in the comfort of God's hands. I spent the night massaging my belly, occasionally singing to her, professing my maternal love to her. From pure emotional exhaustion there were minutes I slept on and off, but I was mostly awake, not wanting to miss a second of the time I had remaining with my daughter.

Morning came and the next step in the process began. It was the beginning of the end. The seaweed had worked. My cervix was dilated and they began the oxytocin. It was our own private D-day. As the contractions began to get severe, I gratefully accepted an epidural. I knew she was small, but having not passed anything that large through my vaginal opening before, I wasn't sure what to expect. Considering all the emotional trauma, I had enough pain to deal with.

The nurses checked me throughout the day and I suddenly dilated very fast. So quickly, in fact, that at one point I had to literally hold my legs closed and wait for Dr. Cohen to come into the room to deliver her. With one simple push our little baby girl came right out. In traditional fashion, Kevin cut the umbilical cord, but that was the only thing that seemed conventional that day. There was no sound of a healthy scream. No rushing to get her cleaned off. No APGAR score. Dr. Cohen gently put her on my chest. Tears poured down my cheeks as Kevin and I took turns cuddling her. It was January 12, 2006, at seven twenty p.m.

I was mesmerized by how beautiful and precious she was. She was indeed tiny, but she was absolutely perfect. She resembled Tyler. She even had his hands. There were dark marks, probably bruising, on her head, which made me wonder whether those were signs of severe brain damage. Her skin was nearly translucent, and I was hypnotized by how delicate and pure this angel looked. Gently and quietly, she breathed soft, subtle breaths.

Her miniature but capable hand gripped Kevin's finger firmly. It was as if she knew her daddy and she was holding on as steadfastly as she could. As we passed her back and forth, she renewed her grip on our fingers, barely able to wrap her hand halfway around, but never letting go. I stared intently at her face, her eyes not yet able to open. *Trust me, baby girl, I don't want to let go either.*

This was one of those moments in time when you have no words to describe how you feel. To acknowledge that you are holding your living, breathing child, knowing that soon she will pass on—and it is totally out of your control. Our decision to let nature take its course had solidified her fate. The amniotic sea within me, meant to shelter her from storms of the outside world, had erupted and forced her to her death. No doctor would rush in and attempt to perform a medical miracle. No amount of prayer to God would change her path.

In the meantime my blood pressure had begun to drop. Dr. Cohen worked to help me deliver the placenta, which I was struggling to do, and massaged my belly as I wrestled to get the afterbirth out. Kevin told me later that the room got very serious as my blood pressure fell lower and lower. Dr. Cohen worked feverishly, and Kevin said my face became ghostly pale. He knew something was wrong. After spending thousands of hours in operating rooms all over the country, he could detect when there was a problem.

Dr. Cohen said firmly to the nurse, "Take her to room one, stat."

Then he turned to Kevin. "She's going to be fine, but there's a little bleeding, and she's having a hard time delivering the placenta. I need some different tools to do what I need to do."

They wheeled me off to the operating room and handed the baby over to Kevin. Here is his account of those very intense moments:

My world came to a crashing halt. I was left holding a dying baby, my wife rushed off to the operating room, unsure of her fate. Was I losing them both today? Only a minute after Stacey was taken out, a nurse escorted a priest into the room and he sat down next to me and began speaking softly. I knew he was making an attempt to comfort me, but my brain was not hearing or processing the words. In fact, I couldn't recollect a single thing the man said. As I sat there I wondered, Are you here for my baby or for my wife? I wasn't even sure—had I uttered those words aloud to the priest? Regardless, he stayed with me the entire time Stacey was in the operating room. I think he and the nurses were afraid to leave me alone. I can easily describe it as the longest and most miserable time of my life…pure numbness.

The baby's movements began to cease. She had been stirring and gripping my finger firmly. But slowly she stopped shifting around. As I held our daughter, she peacefully died in my arms.

That quickly, she was gone.

I sat there clutching our baby. After a while they brought Stacey back to our room. I felt great relief to see her, but I didn't have the words or emotional ability to tell her we had already lost our little girl. I wasn't sure that in that moment she was ready to process the loss of our newest angel.

❧

I was returned to my room, finally free of my placenta and the burden it caused me. I was physically and emotionally exhausted, but still somehow very alert. I wanted to be with our baby.

I was surprised to see a priest waiting in the room with Kevin. He introduced himself to me and asked whether we would like to baptize her. We both instantly said yes, and he promptly removed a seashell from his bag. He asked whether we would mind if he collected some of our tears to use for her baptism, and after we agreed, he gently pressed the seashell against our cheeks and gathered the tears rolling down them, which had not ceased since her birth. As he looked up at us, he asked whether we had given her a name. Kevin and I gave each other one look. Of course we had not discussed a final name. This delivery was completely unanticipated, so nothing had been decided.

And yet without pause, the two of us simultaneously said, "Tess," and smiled. Somehow it seemed just right for her. Our angel Tess. She would be the fifth angel to join our others in heaven.

He proceeded to baptize our little girl, Tess. While I appreciate the formality of the act, I must say that I personally believe all prematurely born or miscarried babies are in heaven, even the ones who don't get the chance to be baptized. I just think God has a place for them there. I think there are circumstances on earth that prevent baptisms from occurring, and God wouldn't hold it against an angel baby and keep him/her from entering the pearly gates. Let's hope I have the chance to find out.

I did not realize yet that she had passed. While she was alive, her breathing had been so slow and subtle it was barely perceptible. It was ten years later that Kevin eventually explained to me when she died. It took me that long to have the strength to ask him about her actual time of death. Quite honestly, this is what my heart and brain processed at that moment: I wanted her to live so badly, and yet the expectation was that she would not survive for long. So the transition between life and death for me with her almost didn't matter. I wanted to hold her and be with her as long as possible in life and in spirit.

For the remainder of the night, Kevin and I took turns holding her and caressing her. We must have told her a thousand times how we loved her.

Kevin left the room on and off to use the bathroom or speak to a nurse. Alone with Tess, I whispered to her how sorry I was that I let her down. How sorry I was that my body wasn't good enough. I told her that I tried my best and that I loved her so dearly. I told her how lucky I was to be her mommy, how beautiful she was, and how much joy she had given me in our short time together. I told her she had a family who loved her and had been praying for her, who wished they could meet her. I told her that one day I'd see her again, and we'd get to spend lots of time together.

Yes, strange as it sounds, I told all of this to my already dead baby girl. How could I not tell her? It might be the only chance I had to let her know how I felt.

The staff at Northside Hospital allowed us ample time with her. They were truly wonderful. Kevin and I called my parents and asked whether they wanted to come in to see her before they took Tess away. Our dear friends and neighbors Lori and Dan Harmeyer were kind enough to go stay with Tyler at the house while he slept. The Harmeyers were like family to us. Tyler referred to them as Mama Lori and Uncle Dan, so I knew that if he awoke he would be at ease with their unexpected presence.

When my parents arrived, they were surprised to see Tess's tiny frame. She was only ten and a half inches long and weighed a mere twelve ounces. As my father held the baby he began to cry, which was unusual for him. It was the kind of cry that was controlled, but his shoulders shook the littlest bit. It felt strange for me, being unable to comfort him, and being the indirect cause of his and everybody else's pain. If my body had just done what it was supposed to, we would not all be here in this predicament.

My parents were grateful for asking them to come. I wish Kevin's parents had been able to be there as well, but that was not possible with their living in New York. When I look back on that night, my only regret was that I did not call Allison to see whether she wanted to visit with us in the hospital; I considered it at the time, but it was so late that night, and it had been such a long day. And it was all so sad. Unsure whether she wanted that degree of sadness while she was pregnant, I felt awkward asking someone, even one of my dearest friends, whether she wanted to come see our dead baby girl. But now I wish I had given her the choice. She could have handled it, and it's something special we could have shared together, brief and odd as it may have been.

Sometime after midnight the hospital staff finally asked whether we were ready to say good-bye to Tess, and we eventually conceded. Pulling her away from us was no easy task; although we readily turned her over physically, it was emotional torture. Even though she had died, the act of letting go was harder than I had anticipated. *Pull it together. You have another child waiting for you at home. Get your act together, Stacey.*

I tried moving my mind to the practical, decision-making aspect of losing her. We had been asked what we wanted to do with her body. Did we plan to bury her or cremate her? Our answer determined what they did with her next. I went to sleep fraught with the events of the day, and the decisions that lay ahead of us in the morning. Kevin slept at home that night so he could spend some time with Tyler when he awoke. We knew it would be a treacherous few days ahead.

THIRTEEN

COPING AND THE
KINDNESS OF OTHERS

When I awoke, my eyes ached as much as my heart. I tried to process the incidents of the day before in my head, and all too quickly I knew it was not just a horrible nightmare, but very much my current reality. I had the nuisance of heavy bleeding between my legs to remind me of that, along with the sights and sounds of my hospital room.

Kevin arrived early that morning, and we were once again offered the chance to hold Tess. Her frail body was cold from refrigeration, but if that was how we had to see her, that was how we'd take her. There is a benevolent group of women in the Atlanta area, the Atlanta Smocking Guild, who donate hand-sewn baptism gowns made for the premature babies born at Northside Hospital. They had dressed Tess the day before in one of these gowns and she was in one again today. It touched our hearts to see that total strangers went to such lengths and had such compassion for families like ours that they would spend hours making these gowns. They were meticulously sewn and smaller than what would fit on most baby dolls. I made a mental note to later thank the ladies who put such effort into making those clothes.

As we held Tess for the last time, we tidied up the loose ends of our stay at the hospital. We told the hospital staff we'd decided to cremate her, and made the appropriate plans to do so. God bless Kevin for managing that. He totally took over, and I am forever thankful that I did not have to deal with those logistics. The nurses gave us her handprints and foot-prints, along with the seashell the priest had used during her baptism. They gave us her baptism gown, and a signed card that read:

> *"In a moment, you and your little one touched our hearts...and though you must travel a lonely, grief-filled road for a while, we want you to know we hold you in our thoughts."*

We were also offered pictures of Tess on a CD. Thank goodness the hospital had a photographer on hand, and the sense to know we would later want images of her. We were so preoccupied with holding our daughter. With the exception of Kevin's cell phone, we didn't have any real camera with us. Kevin snapped a few images, but they were grainy at best. One of them was of Tess grabbing hold of Kevin's finger, clinging to him in her last moments here on earth with us. Her little arm was swallowed by the enormous sleeve of her gown, but her hand poked out and held steadfastly to Kevin's. Her miniature fingers barely covered the top of his index finger.

The Northside Hospital staff had done everything they could to help us adapt to our circumstances. I credit the Perinatal Loss office at Northside for training their staff in how to handle cases like ours. They go above and beyond the call of duty to acknowledge the baby and help you begin the healing process. My three best friends from college asked what they could do after Tess died, and I suggested they make a donation to the Perinatal Loss Endowment Fund. That special group at Northside Hospital is now called the H.E.A.R.T.strings Peri-natal Bereavement Office. In more recent years, they have continued to expand their services, offering a variety of support groups, a newsletter, online resources, a blog, and numerous keepsakes to honor a child who has passed. For me, there was tremendous comfort in reading words shared by others who had written poems or letters of their loss. These pieces were published on their Web site and in their newsletter, and it was an immediate way for me to connect to other bereaved parents. It helped me realize there were other families who had walked in our shoes, and I was not as alone as I felt.

Finally we said our last farewell to our little girl, Tess. She was forever gone but will never be forgotten. The tears started again, but this time there were not as many. My body's water supply had run dry.

My return home was a strange one. It began with a wheelchair ride from my hospital room to the lobby doors of the building. Escorted through the hallways and out to the car where Kevin awaited me, I remembered what it was like bringing Tyler home. That memory worsened the awkwardness of this moment, when my childless arms lay empty. There was no worry about getting our baby properly buckled into a car seat, no introduction of Tyler to his sister, no climbing into the backseat of the car for the ride home to make certain the baby was fine in those first few minutes away from the safety of the hospital. Kevin and I traveled in silence until we walked through the door of our house, where Tyler greeted us enthusiastically. The biggest blessing amid our pain was Tyler, who kept things the slightest bit "normal," if that's what you could call it, for the months I grieved so heavily over the loss of Tess.

On the second day home, my mother took Tyler and me on an errand. Tyler was strapped into his car seat in the back, and I was in the passenger seat in the front, not yet ready to drive.

Tyler peeked around at me. His voice was tentative as he asked, "Mommy, is the baby in your belly all gone?"

"Yes, sweetie. I'm sorry. She is." The tears welled up in my eyes, as my mother pulled out of the driveway.

He seemed just fine with that simple and succinct answer. He didn't look for further explanation or details as to why. For now, that was enough. Tyler was only two years old. I would explain more to him when he was older, or when he sought more information.

There were other aspects of losing Tess that were difficult too—starting with the physical ones that mothers go through. My breasts got tremendously engorged with milk. I was ready to feed what felt like an army of babies…but there was no one to nurse. I was practically screaming in agony. I called Dr. Cohen and pleaded with him to see whether there was any solution for my bountiful (rock-solid) breasts. He suggested placing raw cabbage leaves on them, secured tightly by a bra. I'm not sure how many of you out there reading this have had a similar experience, but overly engorged breasts are no joke. They ache constantly, and when they get touched even the tiniest bit, the pain is what I imagine men would compare to getting hit hard in the testicles. I was in excruciating physical discomfort. While the cabbage-leaf trick may help some, it provided no relief to me.

And, of course, there was the hassle of postpartum bleeding. As if the pain in my heart weren't enough of a reminder, there was the nuisance of managing a heavy period that wasn't balanced by the bliss of caring for a newborn.

In terms of the emotional difficulties surrounding our loss, there were plenty. Most frustrating were the numerous people who asked questions about the baby because they noticed I was not pregnant anymore. Innocently, they didn't put two and two together to figure out that I'd lost her (not their fault…they truly meant well). We faced a plethora of uncomfortable issues, only exaggerated by the fact that our loss was later in gestation.

Not many days after Tess's birth, my father drove Kevin to the crematorium. Kevin remembers the experience well:

> *The drive to the funeral home was surreal. Lee drove as we sat in the car together in complete silence. There were no words to be spoken as we made the journey to pick up Tess's ashes.*
>
> *I remember staring out the window for the half-hour drive as the world passed us by. I was frozen in grief, and time became irrelevant...almost nonexistent. It felt like I was stuck in a terrible dream, one that I couldn't wake up from.*
>
> *The reality of it all became clear again as I stepped out of the car into the funeral home parking lot. I remember taking several deep breaths to ready myself as I waited for Lee to lock the doors and walk over to join me. We looked at each other as if to say,* Well, here we are. This is something we must do. *My father-in-law put his hand on my shoulder as he quietly led me to pick up my only daughter's, his only granddaughter's, ashes.*
>
> *While I don't remember much about our experience in the funeral home, I do recall that the gentleman who assisted us was remarkably kind and compassionate. I had a sense that even for him, there was something extraordinarily solemn about handing over a baby's ashes.*
>
> *He gave me a small envelope with a few documents. Next—at this I was almost in disbelief—he*

carefully handed me a tiny white plastic box measuring two by two by five inches. This container that fit in the palm of my hand held our little girl's remains. It was yet another reflection of her untimely passing.

I thanked him, and then together Lee and I got back in his car to begin the short drive home. It was similar to the drive there. We drove in total silence as I stared out the window and contemplated the gravity of it all.

It was one of the few moments in my life that caused me to question my faith. Why was this happening to me? Why was I going to a funeral home to pick up my newborn daughter's ashes? Wasn't I supposed to die before my children? What had we done to deserve this? It would take years for me to reconcile that I was never in control and that it was all part of God's divine plan for us. It was in that realization that I would eventually find peace.

I was so appreciative that Kevin and my dad completed that task. When Kevin arrived back to our house he handed me a tiny box. Our baby girl was in minuscule particles, much like she was when her life first began. Kevin put her in our safe —truly "safekeeping" for our little angel. We had some ideas about where to spread her ashes, but didn't want to rush into anything.

As the days and weeks after her death passed by, there was one particularly unique and touching gift we were given to honor Tess's short life. It came from Kevin's best childhood friend, Eric, and his wife, Bella. They live in the United Kingdom, and although we don't get to see them often, our relationship remains close. In the spirit of her memory, they arranged to get a star named after Tess. Along with the official certificate was included a map of the star's location. We were so amazed by the thoughtfulness of this gift. It meant that every time one of us looked into the night sky, we would be able to remember her. What a treasure beyond words to have such a special recognition of her time on this earth.

Other friends performed tremendous acts of kindness as well. We received an abundance of handwritten notes, each of which I have kept and read numerous times. There were some who had their churches recognize her loss, or say a Mass in her honor. Another friend made a donation in honor of Tess to Compassion International. Our next-door neighbor and good friend gathered money from additional neighborhood families and gave a donation to the MAMA Project, Inc. (www.mama-project.org). They are a group of people who advocate for severely malnourished children. The loss of Tess inspired others to help children in need.

Each of these gestures and gifts was an expression of love and deep compassion. That support was crucial to my getting through the first few months after her loss.

In the weeks that followed her death, I became something of a robot. My movements were automatic and surreal, almost out-of-body-like. I operated in survival mode. Slowly my grief turned to animosity, as I became frustrated with Tess's absence. Cleaning out the few baby items I had was a chore. *What's the use in keeping them? There's no baby here!* Given that I'd had so many miscarriages, and now with the loss of Tess so late in gestation, I didn't know whether I would ever be able to carry a baby again.

The crib I had been saving for her I decided to go ahead and pass down to my brother and sister-in-law. I gave away a few precious little dresses I had purchased only one week before losing Tess. Ironically, I had been so conscientious to wait to buy them, knowing that I had lost other advanced pregnancies. At twenty-one weeks along, I was certain this time would be different. Surely it was "safe" to start buying just a few small things here and there. How wrong I had been. That made me angry and depressed. I fluctuated between the two.

I was left feeling emotionally raw. Grief is a complex beast to understand. I decided then that time was healing only in that it gives you a chance to figure out how to better manage your grief. It doesn't erase the heartache. The loss of a child and the sadness that accompanies it is a permanent condition. Things I had found easy pleasure in doing before losing Tess left me feeling empty and unsatisfied. I was once unaware of the darker side of life. My old life was one that hadn't witnessed the death of my child, and I yearned to have that back. I didn't welcome my new normal. A number of people told me, "Don't worry—everything will be okay," and hearing that infuriated me. It would never be okay. How could they say such a thing?

Suddenly my own tragedy made me more sensitive to anyone else's pain for whatever reason—loss of a baby, financial ruin, relational distress, a cancer diagnosis, prolonged unemployment. I felt foolish having lived naively for so long. As a person who was historically optimistic about life, I found myself skeptical of the future and wondered whether I would ever be truly happy again. I didn't trust God or anyone else that it would. My old life of innocence was bliss compared to how I felt now. I was consumed with bitterness, anger, and disappointment.

On the few occasions I could muster a smile, it was a false happiness. That mask covered my true feelings, and I used it as a coping mechanism to get through the day. I certainly didn't want Tyler to suffer what I was experiencing, and I tried my best to present a world full of hope for him. He didn't deserve to know that at times life could be this cruel.

One of my most difficult days was when I began to go out on my own again with Tyler. On a weekday afternoon I took him to a local mall in Alpharetta. He loved playing on an indoor playground that was designed specifically for young children. As I entered the playground the hair stood up on the back of my neck. There were women with toddlers and infants everywhere around me. Tyler eagerly ran into the play area as usual, unaware of my growing discomfort.

I took a seat that allowed me to keep a close eye on him. As the minutes passed, a woman and her newborn sat down right beside me. She began to breast-feed her child. My wounds were still too fresh, and I went into a full-on outright ugly cry, with a runny nose and everything, tears streaming down my face. I am certain the people around me wondered what was wrong. I didn't want to say anything to the woman beside me, because I didn't want to make her feel bad for sitting next to me. I knew this public breakdown was bound to happen…I just hadn't been sure when it was going to occur. At least it was among strangers, and I was likely never to see any of these people again. Luckily, Tyler was oblivious to the severity of my meltdown, and I regained control by the time he ran back over to me.

In a weird way, it felt good to have that public-breakdown episode behind me. Getting past it—or better yet, surviving it—made me feel stronger.

FOURTEEN

LETTERS FROM TIM

When I was growing up, we had several dear family friends with whom we spent most of our time. We shared dinners, special occasions, and holidays. Now that many of the families have left Hilton Head and live elsewhere, the group made up of my parents and friends their age still gather for reunions once a year. They call themselves the "Big Chillers," a reference from the iconic movie *The Big Chill*, where old friends come together for a weekend to honor the loss of one of their own. My generation is known as the "Little Chillers," and we now have a third generation forming that has earned the title of "Chillettes." Some of my fondest memories include the times spent with these families. Raising my children in a similar small-town environment with close friends is one of the ways I am trying to repeat this unique experience I had growing up.

When we lost Tess, I sent a brief e-mail to the Big

Chillers. They honored Tess at the Children's Memorial Garden at Hilton Head Island Hospital. In a pleasant setting under a canopy lies a brick bearing her name.

One particular Big Chiller of note was Timothy Coke Doughtie. Tim and his beautiful wife, Betsy, had one son who was fairly close to my age. As a kid, I was fortunate to carpool with their family. It meant extra time with the humorous Tim Doughtie, who was an advertising executive and marketing guru on the island. Hilton Head, as I discussed earlier, was a small community, and Tim had a gargantuan personality. Despite his being a U.S. Air Force veteran, his uniform at that time was a Hawaiian-themed shirt with a casual pair of shorts and sneakers. His characteristic balding head was contrasted by a prominent goatee. This iconic image of his face even graced his stationery. Tim had a deep voice, perfect for radio and television broadcasting, and he could easily transition it into a Daffy Duck impersonation. He made the local news for little tidbits like his quirky musical group, the Phart-O-Phonics (a "classical gas wind ensemble"), and was on a network television show with videos of their family dog, Rumples, a surfing basset hound. Tim owned and operated a comedic T-shirt company, known for their witty sayings. On Hilton Head Island he served on various boards that touched many aspects of the island's growth as a community. The island's hospital board, Community Foundation board, the Island School Council, and the board of hospice care were just a few of the things he dabbled in. His good humor and antics made him extraordinarily skillful at helping to raise money for our community. As a child, I heard many tales of Tim's wild boarding-school pranks that would leave me nearly in tears from laughter.

Tim also had a serious, spiritual side when needed, which I was fortunate to discover. He was a master craftsman when it came to writing, regardless of the subject matter. He had written numerous letters to me while I was on bed rest with Tyler. They were funny and lighthearted, helping me get through those treacherous few months. He always referred to Tyler in utero as "Macho Gazpacho," in honor of his Hispanic heritage.

He sent a similar series of letters to Kevin and me after the loss of Tess. They served as one of the most healing and touching aspects of my grieving and recovery process. After my first e-mail notifying the Big Chillers, I received this short, but sweet note in the mail:

Dearest Stacey:

> *I couldn't let it go without saying.*
> *Your e-mail to the Big Chillers brought tears to my eyes. Your beautiful description connected all of us in such a remarkable way. For you to take the time to share with us this incredibly personal and intimate moment and the reflections of your sadness was an extraordinary gift. One that I will cherish forever.*

My love to you, Kevin, and Tyler.
Tim

His next letter to me was even more remarkable. His note helped put into words the explanation I had been searching for from God as I questioned, *Why* did this happen to us? It's often hard to explain why bad things happen to good people, but Tim was eloquent in his rationale. He helped to provide me with a sense of peace at a time when I needed it most. I wept as I read it.

14 January 2006

Dearest Stacey and Kevin:

> *I can't begin to tell you how I feel. I thought a day or two would give me some clarity to offer you some meaningful comfort. But despite this emptiness I didn't want to just sit here in silence and say nothing.*
>
> *Perhaps if there was a defining moment, it was last night, when the Millers, the Kaplans, the Morgans, Laura and Kyle, and Betsy and I sat around the table with tears in our eyes sharing the pain of it all, each in our own way. There is such a deep, abiding love for you and your family that can only seem to be meaningfully expressed in groups.*
>
> *Your tender embrace of little Tess gave awesome substance to her brief moments here. Surrounded by love, warmth, abundant blessings, and passionate spirituality, she quietly moved on to a better place... never feeling the pains or travails of this world. Such*

compassionate kindness often brings unbelievable sorrow and despair. It is the way.

The great sadness that we all feel is born out of an intense love of promising life and of the belief that good things should happen to good people.

I believe that acts of God and acts of nature are wholly different. Nature rules the random course of things...part of the dynamics God put in place for Creation. God provides all manner of goodness and love. Your time with Tess was a gift of God's assurance that all will be well.

And it will.

With love and heartfelt empathy,
Tim

How perfectly said! It was exactly what I had been searching for. I read the ending again and again:

"...acts of God and acts of nature are wholly different. Nature rules the random course of things...part of the dynamics God put in place for Creation. God provides all manner of goodness and love."

I believe that is one of the most discerning explanations I have ever been given for something so difficult to comprehend. As mentioned, there were times in our stressful baby-making years that I questioned God's existence, or at the very least, my relationship with Him. Was the God I had believed in a trusting and loving God? Recently it didn't feel that way. Tim's words were settling to me. They didn't put an end to the pain, but they did help alleviate some of the anger and doubt I had been feeling. Since we'd lost Tess, my enthusiasm for life had been replaced with uncertainty.

The even more profound part of his letter didn't resonate with me until years later. It was the section where he mentioned that our time with her was a gift, and the assurance that all would be well. I struggled to comprehend how her brief existence would allow me to see that all could be well again. Without question, there was more learning for me to do in that arena.

Tim's outrageous sense of humor combined with his compassionate and deeply spiritual underside were God-given talents. Everyone needs a Tim in his/her life. If only we could all be so lucky.

Kevin and I decided to acknowledge Baby Tess, since we did not plan a funeral for her, by creating a birth and death announcement. I explained to Kevin that I could not handle having a service for her, but I did want to recognize her in some way. A good neighborhood friend of ours ran a home stationery business. She was kind enough to work with me on selecting and printing a card. We mailed it out as we would a birth announcement, but of course, there was the sad news of her passing too. It read:

Please take a moment to remember our little girl
Tess Urrutia
Born and died on January 12, 2006.

She weighed 12 ounces and was 10½ inches.
Although small she was perfect and beautiful.
May our little angel inspire us to count our blessings,
live life with kindness,
and say "I love you" out loud to those we love.
Tess was baptized at Northside Hospital in Atlanta, Georgia.
May she be in peace and watch over us all.
We will never forget her.
Kevin, Stacey, and Tyler Urrutia

Not long after her announcement went out, we received a photo disk from the Perinatal Loss group at Northside Hospital. On the inside of the disk was a note that read:

2/1/06

Stacey,

Your Tess was beautiful. She looks like a little angel. I hope her pictures will bring comfort to you.
Margaret

My sentiments exactly, Margaret. Even the loving eyes of a stranger thought she looked angelic. We welcomed the additional pictures.

Little did I know it, but on that very same day, Tim was busy at his typewriter again. He had received our announcement as well.

1 February 2006

Dear Kevin, Stacey, and Tyler:

> *Your beautiful tribute was divinely inspired.*
> *Tess, this little blithe spirit, touched us all in indescribable ways.*
> *Remembered and cherished.*
> *You will see her in the Sweet By and By!*

Love and consummate peace,
Tim

As time went on, Tim would send us an occasional note letting us know he never forgot us or sweet Tess. The next one read:

Dear Kevin and Stacey:

> *I can't begin to tell you both how much you've been on my mind, in my heart, and in my prayers.*
> *Your odyssey has touched me in incredible ways.*
> *I wish you all manner of good and lovely things.*

Xoxoox,
Tim

There it was again, those words that read, "…all manner

of good and lovely things"—that which I knew he meant only God could provide. How I ached to see the world and my life in that way again. I craved the ability to believe that somehow this would all be okay. That God had a plan for me, and even though I could not understand how he would get me to that happy place once more someday, I wanted so badly to trust that it would indeed happen.

FIFTEEN

CRAZY TRAIN

A couple months after losing Tess, I finally sat down with Kevin to have a serious chat.

I began, "I know it hasn't been very long, but I think we need to talk about how to have another baby."

"Not with this husband," he said quietly but firmly. Kevin couldn't believe what he was hearing.

He continued. "Honey, I love you dearly, but if you ever get pregnant again, it's not going to be with me. We have been blessed with a beautiful baby boy they said we'd never have. He needs his mommy and I need my wife. I am getting off of this crazy train with or without you!"

"Well, here's the deal," I pressed on, the tears rolling down my cheeks. "I know this might sound insane, but I really want another child. I would like to ask you to come explore the options with me. Let's make some appointments with specialists and see what they say about me getting pregnant again, and what our chances are for carrying a baby full-term. Let's take it from there. Let's just hear what they have to say."

Reluctantly he agreed. To be honest, I think he was going through the motions for me. I made the appointments, and soon we were consulting with several physicians who gave us their expert opinion on my ability to carry another baby to term. In short, the answer was not ideal.

We were told that even if I went on bed rest immediately after finding out I was pregnant, which would be mandatory, I would still have only a roughly sixty to seventy-five percent chance of carrying to full term. This would likely mean, of course, taking the necessary medications or steps to get pregnant again, which historically had not been so easy for me. Then hiring someone to replace me as "mom of the house" while I was on full-time bed rest for another eight to nine months. I knew this time around it would not be acceptable to move my mother and/or mother-in-law in for that period of time. So Kevin and I went home to discuss the statistics and scenario we had just been delivered.

He looked at me with an easy conscience, and said with total inflexibility in his voice, "Stacey, my decision is clear. I cannot support your getting pregnant again. You have no idea how scared I was when you delivered Tess. Not only was I distraught that we were losing our little girl that day, but I sat in that room terrified by the notion that I was also losing you. When the priest came into the room as they rushed you away,

I wasn't sure if he was there for Tess or if he was there for you. I refuse to go through that again."

His eyes filled with tears. It was the first time I had any real sense of how panicked he felt that day. I had no concept of how close I had come to my own demise, and he never shared with me the anxiety it had given him.

I respected that, but felt the need to explain to him an equally deep emotion I had.

"Kevin, here's how I see it. I am totally willing to accept the idea that I can no longer carry a baby. It bothers me, but I can accept it. With that said, I can't accept the idea of having only one child in this house. So, you can live with a fairly unhappy wife who has only one child, or we can figure out a way to have another child, and you can have a much happier wife."

There is the familiar saying, "Happy wife, happy life." Well, I normally say, "Happy spouse, happy house," since I feel it should work both ways. In this case, it was not as though one of us was right and the other was wrong. We each had the right to feel the way we did.

Nevertheless, I pressed on. "There are surrogacy and adoption; both are worth considering, and great ways to bring another child into this family. I am content to explore either option. Please think about which one you'd like me to investigate first and that's where I'll start. I feel that strongly about having a sibling for Tyler and, selfishly, another child for us."

Kevin was silent for a moment as he pondered what I said. He was speechless at my persistence to push forward so strongly for another child and probably surprised by how quickly I was eager to move on it. He likes to say that a woman who wants to have a baby is like a runaway train that isn't going to stop until it reaches its destination or has a tragic crash. He felt we were blessed to finally have the one healthy child we did have. Why could I not be satisfied with that? Wasn't one child enough? At least for now?

I tried to explain it further to him.

"I thought that once I had one child, it might be enough. But knowing the joy of one made me want another even more. This is how I have always imagined our family would be. And I just don't feel as though our family is complete without one more child. There are plenty of children out there who need homes, or we can explore the option of surrogacy, which might also be a good choice for us. We are legally more protected in the case of surrogacy, and after the five losses we've had, perhaps it's the right place for us to start."

We had heard of a couple who twice tried to adopt, but for one reason or another it fell through. For other friends of ours, adoption had worked very well. I was eager to take the path of least resistance. A bit of research on surrogacy indicated to me that it might be an easier course. We had experienced enough heartache already.

I begged Kevin, "Please just consider it and let me know how to proceed. But this will be a happier house when there are two children in it." I wondered whether this was how an attorney felt as he tried to argue a case. Perhaps the fact that I was so calm and subtle made my points more pronounced as Kevin listened to my appeal.

"Okay. Start with surrogacy," he conceded.

That was all I needed to hear. I was a girl with a plan. And once again I had a mission.

Kevin thought he was buying time. He was perplexed by my resilience, my continued desire to strive for another child even with everything we had been through. Years later, as we remembered this trying phase of our lives, I would come to realize he was kicking the proverbial can down the road in hopes that my desire would fade away over time and we would move on with our lives.

It was around this time that two events influenced how we each felt about having another child.

First, we received a card from the Perinatal Loss Endowment Fund at Northside Hospital. They sent it intentionally in recognition that it was Tess's original due date, and they had not forgotten. The card read:

The morning glory that blooms for an hour
delights the heart no less than the pine that lives
for a thousand years.

I was incredibly touched. Virtually no one else had remembered this day and the significance it had for us. I thought of Tess every day, and now, four months later, I had gotten to a point where on most days I was able to remember her without tears. This note made me cry like a baby. It all felt so fresh again. Undeterred by my pain, I still longed for another child to share our life with. This acknowledgment of Tess's short life boosted my confidence that I was pushing for the right thing. After reading the card, I gathered my composure and refocused my mind on my husband's new agreement to pursue surrogacy.

The second incident that occurred helped create a change of heart for Kevin. A simple campout with his son opened his eyes to how important his role was as a father:

It was the fall of 2006, and Tyler and I were embarking on our first camping trip. We were venturing out into the great wilds of our pristine backyard in Alpharetta, Georgia. Tyler had just turned three years old, and it was a spectacular setting under the stars together. Our yard was a beautiful haven surrounded by an array of birch, maple, cypress, and weeping willow trees, just to name a few. In the center was a baseball diamond-like bright green lawn. It was the perfect spot for our "adventure" tent. We chose not to install the tent fly so that we could stare through the screen ceiling and gaze at the night sky. Inside the tent we had arranged a few blankets, a couple of pillows, and the ever-critical battery-operated lantern.

After I'd chatted with Tyler for a while, he finally agreed to turn off the lantern and spend some time admiring the stars above. Lying there, we began to drift off to sleep. I decided to ask Tyler one more passing question. As I uttered the words, I remember thinking that it was a frivolous question to ask of such a young child. After all, how insightful could his answer be?

Nonetheless, my words escaped reason and I softly whispered my silly little question.

"Tyler, what do you want to be when you grow up?"

He was snuggled under my right arm, with his tiny head resting on my shoulder. He slowly turned his head toward me with a look on his face that indicated he was surprised I didn't already know.

He answered, "I want to be a daddy just like you." And with that he hugged me tighter. He peacefully closed his eyes and resumed his sleeping position. I could feel his ultimate sense of contentment. Needless to say, my eyes welled up with tears, and I quietly wiped them away as he fell asleep in my arms.

I was the happiest dad in the world. My three-year-old son had just provided an extraordinarily profound answer to my seemingly pointless question. It made me feel so validated to play this role in his life. I went to sleep praying he would grow up to fulfill his dreams—that he would have the chance to experience the joy of being a father who felt as much love for a child as I did in that moment.

Little did Kevin know that less than two months after reading the letter from the Perinatal Loss group at Northside Hospital, I would be asking him to join me on a lunch date that would change our lives in a way I never imagined.

SIXTEEN

SURROGACY 101 CLASS

The moment Kevin gave me the go-ahead, I continued researching to find out everything I could about surrogacy. I discovered most of my information through a friend of my parents who happened to have recently had twins via a surrogate. She was a wealth of knowledge. While there are an abundance of educational sites available to learn about surrogacy now, she advised me to explore Surrogate Mothers Online, LLC (www.surromomsonline.com, also called SMO). Her last resource for me was the name of an attorney, Sara M. Clay, P.C., who specialized in surrogacy law for the state of Georgia.

On the SMO Web site I was able to read all sorts of general information about surrogacy, and surprisingly I found a part of their Web site had a classified section. It allowed for women looking to become surrogates to post their information, or for intended parents (IPs) like us to do the same. A whole new world opened up to me. For weeks, every night after I put Tyler to bed, I would get online and educate myself about surrogacy. I began to respond to gestational surrogate postings by women who seemed to fit what I imagined our criteria would be. It's tough with just a few lines of text to determine whether you've found the right fit, but it was a start. Through several e-mails back and forth, I eventually narrowed the search down to about twelve phone interviews, and initiated the selection process.

As a backup plan, I went out on a limb and reached out to several friends as potential gestational surrogates. A gestational surrogate means the surrogate mother would carry the baby for us, but would not be genetically related to the child. This is in contrast to a traditional surrogate mother, who both donates her eggs and carries the baby. Kevin and I had proved that we had viable eggs and sperm, so we would act as the "donors" in our case.

I was fortunate to have a few very close and, obviously, very generous friends who actually considered getting involved. One woman was a neighbor who lived only a few houses down. She had easily conceived and carried three children of her own and considered her family complete. I was secretly thrilled at the thought of this. She was part of a lovely family, and I knew she would take outstanding care of her body while pregnant. With her proximity, I would also readily be a part of the numerous doctor appointments and prenatal care. I would be able to bring her meals and help make her life easier while she was carrying our baby. She and her husband were devout

Christians, and I felt their offer to do this was as genuine and heartfelt as could be. My gut told me her children would have understood their decision to do this for us. They would be excited for their mother to participate in this ultimate act of giving to our family. Without getting my hopes too high, I phoned Dr. Cohen, who was still our ob-gyn, to get his thoughts on using her as our surrogate.

One simple fact burst my bubble and eliminated her as a likely option: my friend was forty years old. My doctor wanted a younger surrogate for us, someone in her twenties or, at the oldest, in her early thirties. Dr. Cohen explained to me that as you age, the blood flow to the uterus just isn't as good, and it doesn't make an ideal candidate for a surrogate. He said that if I wasn't able to find someone else after I continued my search for a period of time, perhaps she would be a good solution, but he encouraged me to keep looking. He wanted our baby to have the best possible chance.

Next I approached a dear college friend who I suspected had completed her family as well. She had three children and lived in the Northeast. She was another woman who had conceived easily and carried well. In short, between the geographical distance and some health issues that would only be worsened by pregnancy, she was not a good candidate either. But I was amazed that, regardless of her limitations, her heart would have considered a yes. She is one of the most generous and truly kind people I know. I am always grateful for her friendship.

To both of these women I owe a special thank-you. It is not every day that someone is willing to lend her body for nine months of pregnancy, plus several months leading up to it, enduring shots and other discomforts required to help someone else have a baby. The compassion, tolerance, and love involved in even considering that gift are remarkably admirable.

My search continued online with perfect strangers, and after less than two months I narrowed it down to a young woman who was living in Acworth, Georgia. That was only about an hour's drive for me. Although I had interviewed people in Florida, Nevada, Tennessee, California, and a few other states, the person who intrigued me the most also happened to be the geographically closest candidate. It seemed she might be a good match, so we set up a lunch date. She worked in Marietta, so we picked a spot that was close to her office. We planned to meet the following week. Her name was Ella Henderson.

In the meantime, I called legal counsel Sara Clay and established a rapport with her. She was a phenomenal source of information. She walked me through all the necessary steps required to complete the surrogacy process. There was a specific order in which things were to be done, and knowing that in advance would save me a tremendous amount of headache and time. By June of 2006, I had established a formal relationship with Sara and we were well on our way to getting everything organized for our surrogate journey. Kevin participated only in the background, discussing the various elements of surrogacy as I presented pertinent information to him. I respected the fact that he had been hesitant to push forward in this way, and I took full responsibility for taking us down a path he was somewhat reluctant to pursue.

I learned that selecting our gestational surrogate mother was only a small step in the process. There were so many things to consider that were integral to our relationship with the surrogate and relevant to the structure of the "deal":

- We needed to have a psychological review for all involved (that would include a written test for the surrogate and an oral interview for everyone).

- If we received approval there, that doctor/counselor would recommend to the fertility clinic that we be permitted to proceed with the medical screening of the surrogate.

- Assuming the surrogate passed her medical review, Kevin and I would also have to undergo intense blood work to determine that we were not carriers of any blood-borne infectious diseases that could possibly be transferred from our embryo to the surrogate. After all, we were both considered donors in this process.

- We would need to complete a comprehensive legal contract that needed to be signed prior to our beginning any medical treatment. The execution of this contract was mandatory at our infertility specialist's office. It's done to make sure everyone is in agreement prior to implanting the embryo(s).

- There would need to be a mandatory meeting between the doctor, the surrogate, and the IPs to discuss the many possible scenarios that might occur during pregnancy.

These topics included how to handle multiples, how to manage a baby (or babies) with birth defects, or other, more severe, possibly life-threatening issues. The goal was to be sure everyone was on the same page.

- And last but not least, there was the issue of payment. We learned that surrogates are paid for their monthly "hardship" throughout the pregnancy. Surrogates are typically compensated with an additional stipend for occasions on which they have to undergo a procedure. They also usually receive a standard allowance for maternity clothes.

Kevin and I were expected to pay the infertility office their usual fees. Overall, this was going to be an expensive way to make a baby, but we were willing to accept the costs and fortunate to have the means to do so.

It was important to Kevin and me that we find someone who would agree to *our* terms and go along with what *we* wanted. So if we chose to keep a baby who had a particular defect, then we needed a surrogate who was agreeable to that. On the other hand, if nature got "out of control" and divided one or two embryos into eight, we might all need to be comfortable with the idea of selective reduction if multiple embryos were dangerous to the health of the babies or our surrogate. Quite frankly, I just prayed I was never going to have to make that choice. Our goal was to get one healthy baby.

I began to learn which states were legally considered

"surro-friendly" or not (it varies dramatically from state to state), meaning they had laws allowing it or prohibiting it. Some states were categorized as surro-friendly because they didn't have laws providing clarity in either direction. In 2006 (and also at the time of this book's publication), there was no provision on surrogacy in Georgia state law. So it was to our benefit to select a surrogate from Georgia. If we selected a surrogate from a non-surro-friendly state, it was my under-standing that I could not legally pay the surrogate for her services and there would be no enforceable contract.

Speaking of payment, we chose to investigate the option of finding a surrogate ourselves before we considered hiring outside help. There are agencies that fully handle this assign-ment. For us, the cost savings of selecting a surrogate myself combined with doing my own research and interviews allowed for a thorough and sufficient process. I'm sure there are circumstances that make using an agency an ideal choice. Each IP needs to make his/her own decision. What was most important to me was finding someone who would connect with Kevin and me, treat our baby with respect, and have her heart in this for the right reasons. While it was understandable to pay a surrogate, I found there were some women whose primary reason for surrogacy was to give the gift of life to a family who couldn't accomplish that on their own. If I chose a surrogate who felt compelled to do this for us, it gave me the sense that she would be ultraresponsible while carrying our baby.

SEVENTEEN

THE ULTIMATE GIFT GIVER

Kevin arrived home from one of his usual business trips. He was dressed in scrubs and had just walked through the door. The skin below his eyes was puffy from the long week of travel on the road.

"Hi, sweetie! How was your day?" he asked in his customary fashion as we began to reconnect. He leaned down and gave Tyler a bear hug, while offering me his cheek for a kiss. I waited until he poured himself a glass of chilled white wine, a welcome reprieve from the summer heat.

"I think I found our surrogate." I almost sang out the words. That was not the response he expected.

"Seriously?" Kevin nearly choked on his wine.

"Yes," I said cracking a smile. *You get this girl on a mission and she is unstoppable. Especially when it comes to making a baby,* I joked to myself.

"Next week I'm having lunch with a woman named Ella," I informed him. "She lives in Acworth, Georgia, and she's a potential surrogate I've been communicating with who might be a good match for us."

He knew I had been interviewing candidates, but he had no idea how far into the process I had gotten. Having lost Tess in January of that year, I dedicated the following five months to researching the surrogacy industry. Routinely, I would put Tyler to bed and retreat to Kevin's office, where I communicated online with willing surrogate mothers. My aggressive search had led me to Ella. We had exchanged e-mails for several weeks, and finally made the commitment to meet in person. Knowing Kevin is not one who likes a lot of detail, I had intentionally not been filling him in on the conversations until I had something compelling to report.

"Okay, why don't you meet with her first and let me know what you think of her? I'm on the road all of next week. After you meet her we can talk more about it." I suspect he figured I'd never find a qualified candidate that good, or that fast. I could sense Kevin's apprehension in the matter, especially considering how quickly things were moving along. While he had conceded to my plea to either find a surrogate or adopt, he never imagined that once a decision was made, I would act on it so expeditiously. Despite his hesitation I pushed onward with the pursuit. Selfishly, I wasn't willing to wait for him to enthusiastically embrace the idea. Having his conservative agreement on the matter was all I needed.

A few days later, Ella confirmed that we would meet at a Mexican restaurant for our lunch date. I was a little nervous, because although we were selecting her, she was just as equally selecting us. Our initial decision to choose a surrogate would be largely based on intuition. If she was as good a surrogate as I suspected, there were plenty of other IPs out there looking for people like her. We needed to be two strangers crossing paths at the right place at the right time with the right "feeling" for each other. Only subsequent to that decision could we then initiate the process to make sure she was medically suitable to fulfill the role.

The meeting day arrived. With my hopeful anticipation of what the outcome could be, butterflies fluttered in my stomach and I felt like a schoolgirl about to go on a first date. Tyler remained at home with a babysitter. I didn't want the distraction of a toddler interrupting our discussion. It took me nearly an hour to get to the restaurant, so I had plenty of time during the car ride to review what I planned to ask her. I had no idea what she looked like as my eyes roamed the restaurant searching for her. I had given her a brief description of myself and that was it.

As I contemplated whether each patron could be her, I quickly made eye contact with a woman seated at a nearby table. She stood up and came toward me.

"Stacey?" she asked with a shy, warm smile.

"Ella?" I replied tentatively.

How funny to think about that unconventional introduction. The awkwardness of two strangers who first meet, knowing that if the relationship continues as intended, then someday one woman will deliver the other woman's baby.

We gave each other a hug and almost simultaneously said, "It's nice to meet you!"

She had a friendly, bright demeanor. We sat down and began chatting right away. Ella had two children of her own. During our phone interviews, I'd asked a number of personal questions, so I was familiar with her already. She had a little girl, Nicole, and a boy, Mark. She was a single mom, only twenty-three years old. She originally planned to be a surrogate for a friend who thought she couldn't carry a baby, but then the friend was able to get pregnant and have a baby after all. So, she thought, if she was willing to carry a baby for a friend, why not do the same for a stranger? That very night she posted to surromomsonline.com, and within a day I responded.

Ella was a full-time employee at a company not far from where we met, and she had family in town who supported her decision to become a surrogate. More important, we connected on fundamental issues with respect to prenatal care. I noticed she ordered water for lunch, a healthy decision compared to caffeinated choices. I was firm with her on basic things: no smoking, drinking alcohol, or doing drugs while pregnant; always wearing a seat belt while in a car; eating healthy; getting enough sleep. While it may have been assumed that those were obvious demands of our surrogate, they seemed worth reiterating. We had covered many of these topics on the phone. Seeing her reaction when discussing them in person could provide me with an added sense of security or raise new concerns. It's a line of questioning that some may consider trivial; to me, there was nothing more crucial than understanding the habits of someone who would be carrying our baby.

I was concerned about how tired Ella might become while being pregnant and taking care of two other children, which is draining on anyone. However, in my mind I was already planning out the meals I could deliver on a weekly basis in an effort to make her life easier. The Helping Hands group in my neighborhood had made my life more manageable during an exhausting time; shouldn't I do the same for her?

Ella seemed comfortable with everything we discussed, including the idea of taking all the shots necessary for the surrogacy process to work. With rush-hour traffic, it would be logistically next to impossible for me to drive to her to administer injections every day post-implantation of the embryo(s), so she would need a friend or relative who was comfortable helping her. She said she had a person in mind who would be perfect for the job. That friend happened to be a phlebotomist, who would be competent with the use of needles.

Last, and perhaps most important, she reassured me that at the end of the day, this would be our baby, not hers. She agreed that if at any point along the way a decision regarding the health of the baby had to be made, it would be our decision. She added that if the roles were reversed, she would want the same parental authority herself.

She asked me about our family and our pregnancy history, and I told her our story. By the end of lunch we had covered a lot, and it was time for her to return to work. We left the meeting deciding that a good next step would be for each of us to go home and think about what we had discussed and get back to each other. I needed to debrief with Kevin. He's great at reading people. I knew that if I had done a good job with the initial screening, he could help me with a final selection on the "trustworthiness" factor. I tend to give people the benefit of the doubt, and I am admittedly somewhat gullible. Kevin has lots of experience with interviewing candidates for jobs, and can more readily detect when people are misrepresenting themselves. I wanted him to meet Ella… assuming she liked me enough to go forward.

Later that evening, Kevin and I had the chance to talk once Tyler was in bed. I shared with him the events of the day and, in particular, my very special lunch date. I encouraged him to consider her as a very real candidate. Kevin was flabbergasted, shocked that I actually found someone who fit the criteria I was looking for to be our surrogate mother, and had done it so swiftly.

I defended my actions. "Well, you gave me a goal of finding a surrogate, so I went to work on it. And I didn't waste any time. I think you'll really like her. I'd love for you to meet her and give me your opinion, assuming she liked me as much as I liked her. So, what do you think?"

I waited tensely for him to respond.

"Okay, sure. Sounds good to me," was all he could say. I had, after all, performed the appropriate background research to confirm that we were selecting the right person. Kevin's lack of enthusiasm didn't persuade me to slow down the process. I was starting to figure out that if we were to have another child, I would need to take the lead. I would rely on his support and participation some times more than others, but in general, I didn't need him to be as involved in the process, strategically or medically. I made the following conclusion: Kevin could take a backseat role as long as he was emotionally happy with the end result—a baby. With that one concession I could continue to push the process forward.

Now all that was left was a meeting between Kevin and Ella.

"Oh, yeah, one more thing I should probably tell you before you meet her," I said. "Ella happens to be black."

"Really? Where's the hidden camera?" he joked as he absorbed the news. "I guess I never even pictured a woman who didn't look like you, whether she be African-American, Asian, or Hispanic. As long as she's the right person to carry our baby, and assuming I like her as much as you do, I'm fine having her as our surrogate," he said casually, just as I thought he would.

I found the level of surprise slightly ironic coming from him. I had, after all, chosen to marry Kevin, who was Cuban. If I chose a Hispanic spouse, why wouldn't I have considered other races for our surrogate mother? At the time, Kevin's sister was married to a black man, and together they had a beautiful little girl, our beloved niece. Our family was a melting pot of sorts. Ella would fit right in.

As for me, our race differences were a nonissue. My parents are some of the most loving and generous people I know, so between their unprejudiced way of living and the reinforcement of growing up with prominent black leaders in our community, I was raised to believe all people are created equal. In our house we didn't define people by their skin color but rather by the quality and content of their character.

I mentioned Ella's ethnicity to Kevin because I felt certain that having this communion of sorts would not be entirely popular in the Southeastern United States. I wanted to make sure he was ready for that should anyone dare to make an uncalled-for comment. Since he'd grown up in New York City, it was more common for him to see interracial couples or hear of blended families. In the South, this could get people's attention, and I wanted him to be ready for remarks or stares we might get as a result of our choice. Kevin was thick-skinned and undeterred, so we easily made the decision to move forward with considering Ella as our surrogate. She didn't imply that our contrasting race was the least bit of an issue for her either; in fact, we never once discussed it. Her impartial and unbiased attitude was another thing I admired about her.

Shortly after our first acquaintance, Ella and I were back in touch. We both agreed it had been a good meeting, and we wanted to proceed. We made plans to have lunch again, and for Kevin to join us this time around. Only a few days later the three of us gathered at the same Mexican restaurant where she and I first met (I quickly learned it was Ella's favorite spot).

Our session this go-around was equally as friendly and comfortable as the first. Kevin and Ella took the opportunity to get familiar with each other. The conversation flowed easily between them, and at the end of the meal we departed with hugs. We once again decided to mull things over and talk in a few days.

The moment we were in the privacy of our car I looked over at Kevin with excitement.

I didn't waste any time. "So, what did you think?"

"I agree," he admitted. "She seems like a great fit. I think you made a good choice. I like her, and you know I tend to go with my gut when I meet people."

"Well, let's see what she thinks of us after meeting you," I said, teasing him now that she'd had the chance to interview both of us. I felt quite certain our time together would only have improved our chances that she would be willing to act as our surrogate. Nevertheless, I was still keeping my fingers crossed and saying my prayers, not taking a thing for granted.

On the car ride home Kevin reached over and held my hand, squeezing it firmly. I knew my husband well, and subtle as this gesture might be, it was his way of indicating that he was satisfied not only with our choice to use Ella, but in general in with our decision to use a surrogate.

Sure enough, only a few days later, when Ella and I touched base, we agreed we were still interested in moving forward together with the process.

This was where the real planning began. Our first step was the interview with a counselor or psychologist, which was much more of a burden on Ella than on us. She had to take a long written evaluation to basically confirm that she wasn't a deranged woman entering into an unhealthy arrangement.

After her written exam, the three of us had individual and group psychotherapy sessions with our counselor. The sessions were extensive dialogues about how we each felt about the surrogacy. Ella met with the therapist one-on-one, and

Kevin and I met with her as a couple. Then all three of us met with her together. We all hoped this went well, because if we did not pass any portion of the interview we could not move forward with the medical component of the surrogacy. Though the evaluations were time-consuming, I admit they were an important part of the process, because for IPs and surrogates who are not in sync, this conversation is an effective technique for bringing up any undisclosed topics, feelings, or concerns. During our time together so far, we had gone over so many of the discussion points already, there weren't any surprises. In my opinion, the consultations went smoothly.

Fortunately the counselor agreed, and within a week she sent a letter of recommendation off to both attorney Sara Clay and Dr. Goldsmith (our reproductive endocrinologist at the infertility clinic). Thank goodness for Ella's sake there was no need for a repeat or second opinion—her evaluation had really been a long day for her, and surely an exhausting one. Had the session not gone well, it would mean repeating the process with a different counselor or, worst-case scenario, our finding a new surrogate.

The next step was to begin a basic medical workup on Ella with regard to her fertility health. Around the same time, they drew blood from Kevin and me and sent it off to a special lab (to the tune of several thousand dollars per person) to screen for any blood-borne pathogens, sexually transmitted diseases, or any other infectious diseases that Kevin or I might be able to transfer to Ella via our embryo. As donors, we were under tremendous scrutiny, and rightfully so. We received good news all the way around. Ella had good uterine/general health, while Kevin and I were given the all-clear from the lab results to proceed as donors.

We met with Sara Clay to finalize the contract of the surrogacy agreement, which seemed amicable. I'm not sure whether the degree of friendliness we experienced is typical between most surrogates and IPs, but I imagine it is. At this point in the process, everyone is eager to move forward, and both parties are excited to get started. In less than two months after our first meeting we had signed our surrogacy agreement with Ella.

Ella and I then met with Dr. Goldsmith and his staff to commence our medical protocol. There was an elaborate and specific process by which they prepared both Ella, as the surrogate, and me, as the egg donor, to ready us for the embryo transfer. They needed to prep Ella's body, which involved giving her a variety of medications to help prepare her uterus to receive the embryo. Through medications I injected, they increased my egg production and prepared for the retrieval, or harvesting, of my eggs. It all had to be perfectly timed. A "fresh" embryo transfer would be more ideal and would statistically lead to better results, so we aimed to accomplish that. Kevin's sperm was collected and tested ahead of time. The transfer process would be similar to a standard in vitro fertilization procedure, except rather than putting the embryo back into me, they would put it in Ella.

For the next two months, Dr. Goldsmith worked our hormonal calendars into synchrony as described above. He created a medicinal cocktail that readied Ella for implantation and allowed me to produce a surplus of eggs (also called follicles). I gave myself injections religiously, every day as instructed, and went in for multiple ultrasounds and repeated blood work. Ella went in for blood work as well, and anytime she had an appointment I joined her.

It was always a two-for-one special. If they had an appointment for her on the books, they also saw me. I felt it was a chance for us to get to know each other better, and I enjoyed that. It was a little funny being in the infertility office with her. I'm sure people couldn't figure out whether we were partners trying to have a baby or what the deal was, but we were obviously there together.

I'm sparing the details on the specifics regarding our medical workup because there are plenty of medical resources that discuss that element of in vitro fertilization. The regimen we used could be totally up-to-date still or somewhat obsolete, so there is no need to elaborate. As any woman who has been through surrogacy knows, while it seems like a cumbersome and lengthy process at the time, it is a routine that most of us would readily go through again in the attempt to have a child.

As time went by, we each primed our bodies for the transfer. My egg retrieval day finally arrived, and it was the first major medical feat in our transfer process. I was so excited I could barely stand it. I put the discomfort of the procedure out of my head, and welcomed what was about to come. They took my follicles and fertilized them with Kevin's sperm the same day. They allowed the embryos to develop and grow, and only a few days later we were ready for the transfer.

The news was not ideal. While I had produced a decent number of follicles, only one embryo looked really good. All the others either failed or were bad. There is a ranking system the infertility office uses to evaluate the quality of the embryos, and I had only one high-ranking embryo. Eleven oocytes (eggs) were retrieved; seven were mature and fertilized, which ultimately resulted in only three viable embryos. There was an eight-cell, a six-cell, and a four-cell embryo. Dr. Goldsmith suggested we transfer all three embryos, given the unlikelihood that more than one would implant.

The goal we had discussed with Dr. Goldsmith was to have one healthy baby, so I remained optimistic. All we needed was one good embryo. Just one.

There was a different doctor on call the day we performed the transfer of the embryos to Ella. Kevin was on the road for business, so I waited alone while the team prepped her, but the doctor and nurses allowed me in the room for the actual transfer. It was a surprisingly simple procedure, both pain-free and fast. Using a catheter, he easily guided the embryos into her uterus. The doctor could "see" where to place the embryos, since the medical team was using ultrasound. He explained to me that embryos are naturally "sticky," and that the doctor just assists with helping the embryos get to an ideal location in the uterus for implantation. I was fascinated by the whole process.

A familiar thought struck me in that moment: We had attempted to make a baby and Kevin and I hadn't even been in the same room. Was that okay? Was that "acceptable" to God? We had used external measures to conceive Tyler. Here we were doing a similar albeit different version of assisted conception again today. Certainly we would face criticism from others who would not understand. To them I would argue that infertility is a treatable medical condition comparable to cancer or diabetes. Should we not pursue treatment for our diagnosis much like those other patients would? While the traditional act of making love was not being employed, there was still the act of love between Kevin and me, in our desire to bring a baby into this world. Hadn't God created the people who could help us with our problem? I tried reassuring myself. *People who have a difficult time conceiving or carrying have done this countless times before us.* I couldn't fathom a God who would fault me for wanting to be a mother. The amount of time our child would spend in a petri dish, and even in the body of another woman, was infinitesimal compared to the rest of his or her life. Did the mechanism we used to conceive a baby really matter in the grand scheme of things? Wasn't the lifetime of love we could give a son or daughter more important than the road we took to get him/her here? If anything, couples like us who struggled to have a baby valued the miracle of life even more than usual, taking nothing for granted. I continued to contemplate our circumstances as I prayed for the making of a child in that room.

Ella rested comfortably on the table for about ten minutes, and then I gave her a huge hug before she left. I knew that in a matter of about ten days, we would be able to tell from the pee-stick tests whether or not she was pregnant, and the doctor's office would perform a blood test shortly after that to confirm it.

While we were waiting for pregnancy results, Kevin, Tyler and I made a visit to Hilton Head to spend time with my grandmother, my parents, and our Big Chill friends. We gathered together for my grandfather's funeral. His poor health had finally brought his life to an end; thankfully, it had been a peaceful passing. But during our mourning for my grandfather's rather expected departure, we learned Tim Doughtie had been experiencing severe and puzzling issues concerning his health. His condition was declining at an alarming pace, and tests were being done to provide a diagnosis.

It was around this time of uncertainty that I received another letter from Tim. It was waiting in our mailbox when we returned home. The witty, yet poignant card read:

Dear, dear Stacey.

> *What a joy, delight, thrill, and treat to see you and Tyler this weekend! Now, with the miracle of surrogacy fancifully looming in the future, I'd like to place my order: ONE TYLER TO GO.*
> *Without question, that little fellow is one of the most endearing and exceptional kids I've ever met. He defines you and Kevin in remarkable ways. To you both, my compliments!*
> *And as you follow your new pathway, I wish you every moment filled with exuberance and wonderment. What a gift.*
> *As one of your most ardent admirers, I see in you a beautifully defined sense of spirituality and perspective.*

The sadness of late has enriched you in amazing ways. Indeed, yet another gift. This one from your daughter.

Thanks for coming, Stacey. You always bring such goodness.

Love and best to you, Kevin, and my buddy Tyler!

Xoxo,
Tim

Simultaneously it brought tears to my eyes and a smile to my face. He understood the excitement we felt at the anticipation of a baby, and the hope we held in our surrogate. And, oddly, he already recognized one of the many "gifts" I received from Tess that I would only years later begin to comprehend.

Little did I know this would be Tim's final letter to me. Shortly after he crafted it, he received a horrifying diagnosis. Doctors informed him that he had late-stage pancreatic cancer. Just three weeks later, I quickly made another trip from Alpharetta to Hilton Head Island. I understood how rapidly his health was declining, and didn't want another day to go by without telling him in person how very much he'd meant to me in my darkest hour. Tim was in the comfort of his home, already receiving hospice care. In my humble opinion, it was actually a beautiful and peaceful way to die. I give Tim's wife, Betsy, and their son a lot of credit for helping him have the best quality of life he could in his final days here on earth. Their love for him in the home was palpable. Tim was stretched out on a bed in their living room. His view was the serenity of the marshland. Bird feeders were scattered among the trees—a reminder of how alive things were outside his home. The setting was perfectly tranquil, except for the emotional undercurrent coming from me. I greeted Betsy with a warm hug and we spent some time together. I admired her strength. Then, despite her numbered days with the love of her life, she gave me some time alone with Tim.

I began by telling him how much I had enjoyed growing up with him. That I loved his sense of humor and how infectious it was, and how I wished Tyler could have the joy of knowing him for as many years as I did. I told him he was a real gift and a treasure beyond words, and there was no one else just like him. The world was a much better place with Tim Doughtie in it. It didn't seem very fair that God was taking such a great person from us. I thanked him for the letters he had written to me when I was on bed rest with Tyler, and again when we lost Tess. And last, I told him that I loved him, and that when he got to heaven, to please tell my sweet Tess I said hello. I knew he would be a good messenger.

I wasn't sure he heard a word I said. The whole time I spoke to him, I was gently stroking his hair and massaging his arm and back. He was weak and totally unresponsive. His eyes were closed and he was barely breathing. I stood there a few minutes taking in his face, knowing it would be the last time I would see him alive. I decided then that nature and death have something in common: They operate without prejudice. They don't act on a bias of good people versus bad people, and each one of us is susceptible to their attack. Of all people, Tim understood that.

Breaking the silence, he uttered three simple words: "I love you."

Oh, the glory in that moment. He had heard me.

On October 1, 2006, the very same year we lost Tess and my grandfather, we also lost Tim. It had been only one short month since he was diagnosed. It was absolutely heart-breaking not only for his family, but for many. This shocking and unexpectedly quick loss was a painful void for the entire community. I took it especially hard.

It seemed like the longest week and a half of my life. I had the sadness of Tim's departure on my mind, combined with the anxiety of waiting to hear the outcome of our embryo transfer. Finally, nine days after the transfer, Ella texted me with the results. But it was not the news we wanted: Her home pregnancy test was negative. We held out a little bit of hope, thinking that perhaps it was too early to tell. After all, we had never done IVF before. Maybe things were different when implanting a transferred embryo.

The next day I waited with bated breath when the phone rang and the caller ID indicated it was the infertility office. But the news was not good from them either. The pregnancy blood test had also come back negative.

Ugh! How soon can we start a new cycle? I tried to remain calm and remember it often takes more than a single attempt to make an IVF transfer work. Before I got my questions out, the nurse on the line was telling me the plans for when we could begin our next round. I was pleased with that. I had a focus, which was mentally healthy for me. They had already contacted Ella to make sure she agreed with the plan as well. She had been such a trooper to do this once. We were indebted to her, and so thankful she was willing to try again. Ella seemed equally disappointed that the first implantation hadn't taken and was enthusiastic for round two.

Fortunately, within a matter of weeks, we repeated the workup routine. This time we were old pros at taking our meds, and there was a comfortable familiarity to it all. I had to duplicate the egg-retrieval component of the process, because I had no surplus, or remaining embryos, harvested from the last round to use for this transfer.

The workup was seamless, and we once more found ourselves meeting on transfer day. This time Dr. Goldsmith was the doctor performing the procedure. I explained to him that I had given Ella a special necklace my aunt made. On it hung a simple cowry shell, which is often the symbol of womanhood, fertility, and birth. She had made one for each of us, and both Ella and I faithfully wore them throughout our entire workup. Dr. Goldsmith smiled and said he could add a little special something himself. After the transfer was complete, he held his hands in the air above Ella's abdomen and chanted a few words in a language that was not familiar to me. He explained it was something special that he and his young daughter had contrived…their own version of a fertility-inspired mantra. The wording was derived from the Elven language (specifically Sindarin) in J. R. R. Tolkien's book series, *Lord of the Rings*. The origin didn't particularly matter to me. I just liked that he was adding his own element of spirituality to the day's activities. I welcomed any form of prayer or good luck.

I had a positive feeling about this round. I was "cautiously optimistic," as some like to say. Perhaps it was because this time we had slightly better odds going into the transfer. In this second attempt we transferred three embryos, an eight-cell, a seven-cell, and a six-cell, to Ella, again with the hope that only one would implant and give us the child we had been praying for. God and science would figure it out for us. It was in His hands and out of our control. I marveled once more at the fact that Kevin and I didn't need to be in the room together while our embryos were moved to Ella's body. He was out of town for work, but was eager to know how everything had gone. We both had high hopes that this round would be successful.

In addition to the transferred embryos, we had two four-cell embryos remaining that they left for observation in case they continued to grow. They would monitor those embryos for another two days to determine whether they could be frozen for our future use.

I gave Ella a warm hug good-bye and sent her on her way to rest for the day. I thanked her profusely, knowing that the progesterone injections she had to tolerate, at least until a pregnancy test could be administered, would not be fun. She reminded me that they really weren't so bad, and I felt blessed to have found such an amazing partner in our surrogate journey.

We decided to stay in touch as usual, agreeing to pay special attention around day nine, when she would perform an over-the-counter pregnancy test just for our entertainment. The normal waiting time to test for pregnancy was ten to twelve days, at which point the infertility office would evaluate the level of hCG in her blood. As mentioned previously, the hCG level was important—it's the hormone produced during pregnancy that typically doubles about every two or three days —and tells you whether you are pregnant. This time frame for testing is used because home pregnancy tests after IVF may result in false positives and false negatives. In most IVF cases, a false positive can occur because hCG is used to trigger ovulation for the egg retrieval from the mother. This could leave a trace amount of hCG in the mother's bloodstream, thus giving a positive pregnancy result without an actual pregnancy. In our case, because we were using a gestational surrogate, no hCG shot to trigger ovulation was used on Ella, so the detection of any hCG in her blood would be a significant finding. A false negative was also possible, since levels of hCG may not be high enough on the testing date to detect a positive pregnancy result.

I waited on pins and needles as the days slowly passed by. Only a couple days later, we got word from Dr. Goldsmith's nurse that the two additional four-cell embryos were no longer viable. We had no "frozen babies" to think about.

And so we waited....

EIGHTEEN

SOMETIMES IT TAKES THREE

Early on the morning of day nine, Ella got in touch with me. First there was a text reading, "I have good news!" and then we spoke live over the phone. Kevin planted himself next to me while I made the call. My hands shook as I dialed the number. She didn't bother to say hello, as her enthusiasm could not be contained: "It's positive! The test is positive!" She had woken up that morning and peed on a home pregnancy test as her first morning duty.

My jaw practically dropped to the floor and I had a kind of silent-scream reaction. I could tell how genuinely excited she was too. Practically knocking Kevin off the couch, I started jumping up and down and began telling her how great the news was. I quickly settled down and Kevin wrapped me in a bear hug, a grin lighting up his face. Words couldn't describe how elated we felt.

We discussed that she was due for her blood test soon at the doctor's office, but I felt confident that it would only confirm what we had just learned. The next questions were, How many embryos implanted? Was it a viable pregnancy? Would we see a heartbeat and a gestational sac to confirm that within the next two to four weeks?

I didn't mean to rush her off the phone, but I told Ella I needed to go so that Kevin and I could rejoice in the news with our family. It just happened to be Thanksgiving week. What a special thing for us to be thankful for!

The timing was particularly ironic. Only a few years before, we had announced to our family that we were pregnant with our first child, and I had told everyone while gathered together at Thanksgiving. We went on to lose that baby at nearly eighteen weeks' gestation, on my thirtieth birthday. Here we were again at Thanksgiving time, sharing the news that our surrogate was now pregnant with our seventh baby. This time I prayed our outcome would be different. It was our baby, but the woman carrying him/her was hopefully a more suitable specimen than I was for the job. We were counting on this.

Ella followed up at Dr. Goldsmith's office with her blood test, and it was indeed a positive result. Her hCG numbers looked good. The doctor asked her to return in two days in order to repeat the blood work. This would give them an idea whether things were moving along according to plan. It also could indicate whether more than one embryo had implanted, which would be suggested by elevated hCG numbers.

Ella's hCG levels rose normally over the next few days and weeks, indicating that there was just one fetus developing in her uterus. This was a crucial time for Ella's friend to correctly administer the progesterone shots. It would help her retain the pregnancy until her body began producing enough progesterone to function on its own.

Soon it was time for her first ultrasound, and sure enough, things were confirmed as we expected. To our great relief, there was only one fetus present. I felt such excitement at seeing our tiny baby growing inside of Ella, and had enormous hopes that this time we would have a successful outcome.

I remembered thinking to myself that all it took was just one good embryo. It looked like God had granted our wishes. We had a long nine-month wait ahead of us for the final prize, and we were all too aware of the many things that could go wrong along the way. Nevertheless, we were off to a good start!

I marveled at the miracle of what it takes to make a baby and how often it all works "according to plan." There are so many things that can go wrong, and yet so often it all goes right. We are each our own unique phenomenon.

Consider how cells divide to become organs, each of those components acting in concert with other body parts to create a functional human being. It is a system that is extraordinarily complex. To me, it's evidence that there is a God who oversees the intricacies of this process over and over again for the creation of each of us. If you think for a moment about how complicated the development of our hearts, our brains, our intestines, and our vascular system is...just those few constructs of our bodies alone seem impossible to build without defect.

We have, for example, more than sixty thousand miles of vessels in our bodies. Doesn't it seem *something* would go awry along the way? And yet so often it all operates meticulously well. It is a mysterious and almost magical process, one I see as truly divine. To say the least, as a parent who has seen the process fail, I appreciate the miracle of it all, and how very often it leads to a perfect little baby.

Ella went to Dr. Goldsmith for checkups during her first trimester. After that point, and with no reason for concern in the pregnancy, she transitioned to Dr. Cohen's office. He managed her for routine ob-gyn appointments throughout the remainder of the pregnancy. I accompanied her on every doctor visit and we began to get to know each other quite well. With Ella's permission, Tyler often joined us. He understood that Ella was carrying his little brother or sister, and he loved seeing the baby on ultrasound. In simple terms, Kevin and I had explained why his sibling was in another woman's body. I was relieved he didn't ask us any questions, just accepted what he had been told.

Because of my high-risk status in pregnancies prior to this one, Ella was also seen by Dr. Ryan Miller; he was the primary perinatologist I saw during all my previous pregnancy troubles. It was at one appointment with Dr. Miller that Kevin, Tyler, and I attended with Ella that we found out the baby's gender. The ultrasound room was packed with our animated group. I'm sure having so many people invested in the care of one baby was a little odd for Dr. Miller, but he handled it in stride. Ella was predicting that the baby would be a girl, and for that reason I anticipated a girl as well. I also think that because I had planned to bring a girl home when pregnant with Tess, my brain just somehow expected this baby to be a girl too. That was in no way logical or rational, but heightened emotions can erase all logic—and we women can be particularly good at experiencing this.

The ultrasound began and we waited eagerly and a bit anxiously…first to make sure that the baby's overall health was good, and then eventually to find out the gender. I didn't care what the sex of the baby was as long as it was healthy. We had come so far and worked so hard just to get where we were. I was most interested in making sure we heard a strong heartbeat, that the baby had all his/her parts, the organs were functioning well, things of that sort.

Finally we got to the fun stuff, and looked at the baby's "nether regions." The technician asked whether we wanted to know; in unison Kevin, Ella, and I exclaimed a resounding, "Yes!"

As she moved to the area where the baby's genitalia were, Kevin and I looked at each other and said, "It's a boy!" before she could even get the words out.

We had seen so many ultrasounds that we knew right away what boys looked like on ultrasound scans, versus girls. The technician confirmed our guess, and Ella was surprised to hear that everything she had been thinking and feeling with regard to the sex of this baby was different from her prediction.

Tyler beamed, and with a huge grin on his face he quickly asked, "Can we bring him home with us?"

We of course explained to him that the baby needed to finish developing inside of Ella's body for quite some time still. Tyler was just so excited, and pressed again, asking if he could "please, please bring the baby home today?"

In an effort to divert his attention from the subject, we checked out of the office and said our good-byes to Ella. As we made our way out to the car, we talked to Tyler about what he might like to name the baby.

"How about Artie?" he said. Although he was completely serious, Kevin and I couldn't help but ask him to suggest another name.

He thought for a moment, and after some contemplation said, "How about Artie Fisty?"

Kevin and I just cracked up. We couldn't help it.

Kevin said aloud, "Our future child, Artie Fisty Urrutia. I'm not sure about that name, Tyler. We may have to give it a little more thought before we come up with a final name, buddy."

We just chuckled as we got into the car.

"I like it!" Tyler insisted.

"Well, Daddy and I get veto power," I chimed in, "but we'll consider it." It was a happy ride home. One of the best we'd had in a long time. Seeing our baby boy growing so big and healthy on the ultrasound screen was the best gift we could have asked for.

As a means of making her life easier, I would occasionally bring dinner to Ella and her children. I was trying to think of things that would make her day a little bit simpler, anything to lighten her load for the burden she was bearing on our behalf.

It gave me great pleasure to see her looking so healthy, and it was a nice way to drop off her surrogacy payment in person, or just hang out for a while. Ella's children were very sweet. Tyler adored playing with them.

As the months passed, one of the more fun things Ella and I got to do together was go shopping for maternity clothes. While it may not have been my belly that was ever growing, there was still something very satisfying about joining Ella on that shopping trip. Every step along the way meant great progress, and I knew how precious that advancement was. I didn't take anything for granted. I asked my mother to join us on our excursion. The store clerks must've been surprised at how unusually excited we all were to be buying maternity clothes. I'm sure they couldn't figure out exactly what our relationship was, but they picked up on how happy we were that there was a baby on the way, and did everything they could to be extra helpful.

My mother, Ella, and I sat down to have lunch together after the shopping spree was over. As I got up from the table to head for the bathroom, my mom proceeded to thank Ella again for the gift she was giving us. She was curious to know more from Ella. I paused to hear this exchange before walking away.

"I know why Stacey picked you to be her surrogate, but how did you know she was the right person for you?" she asked.

"After I made the posting on surromomsonline.com, I got responses from a number of people looking for a surrogate. There was just something that connected me to Stacey. Even though there were often posts from various people, I would always read Stacey's first," Ella responded.

Funny thing was, I had felt exactly the same way about Ella. We had never talked about why we chose each other. It was just an unspoken kinship between us that, believe it or not, could be felt across the World Wide Web.

One of our more comical moments in the surrogacy process was partway through the pregnancy, when I rented a hospital-grade, top-of-the-line breast pump. For more than a month I tried pumping to get my milk supply going, with the hopes that maybe I would be able to nurse the baby after he was born. I would sit on the couch in our bedroom, with both breasts in the pumping cups and the machine on full throttle.

One particular day, Kevin walked in and gave me a look that indicated that he thought this was a crazy attempt at providing homegrown breast milk for our future child.

I responded to the look with a loud and exuberant, "Mooooooo!" I had breast-fed Tyler for over a year, and I was bound and determined to give this baby the same healthy start I had given our other child.

For Tyler we used to joke that the "breastaurant" was open for business, and depending on which breast he nursed from, there was the option of chocolate or vanilla from the "booby buffet." Tyler was healthy as an ox, and I felt he was that healthy in part because he had been fed breast milk. Despite pumping every three hours like clockwork, I had only a few drops of milk leaking out. And that was after a month of pumping! It was disrupting our summer schedule constantly, and we were forced to break away from all sorts of things to rush back to the house to fit pumping into our daily routine. After a month and a half, and nearly in tears, I called my friend Allison.

She gave me the official "out." As a pediatrician, she swore to me that it would not be the end of the world if I stopped pumping and fed our next baby on formula alone. She explained that if I continued pumping, it was unlikely that I would ever produce enough milk to supply exclusively breast milk. I would need to supplement with formula, which would alter his immune system. Apparently, in laymen's terms, formula alters the gastrointestinal flora and therefore changes the body's reaction to the environment (such as to allergens, bacterial infections, viruses, etc.). Introducing *any* amount of formula would lead to this same result, so torturing my body for a few drops of breast milk each feeding really didn't make sense. She assured me that there were good formulas available on the market that would allow me to raise a healthy baby. I did not need to be the martyr I was turning myself into.

When I told Kevin of my decision to stop pumping, his only comment was, "God bless Allison for talking some sense into you. The Lord knows I couldn't."

As time passed, one of the legal requirements of our surrogacy was an "order of declaratory judgment." This proceeding would give Kevin and me paternity, maternity, and parental rights for our as yet unborn child. Sara Clay, our attorney, had explained early on in our relationship that this was standard procedure in surrogacy agreements. It typically takes place at approximately seven months' gestation (I assume they pick this time frame in case there is a premature birth). One of the benefits of this judgment, assuming all went well, was that we would not need to legally adopt our child after he was born.

We were told it would be an amicable hearing that, from a practical standpoint, would allow Kevin and me to make any and all decisions for the baby the moment he was born. It would also allow for our names to go on the baby's birth certificate as his parents. I worked with Sara and her paralegal to prepare the paperwork for the judgment.

Kevin and I spoke to Sara before the process began. We just weren't sure what to expect.

"What if Ella doesn't agree? What would happen then? How do we handle that?" Kevin asked.

He wanted to feel prepared for any possible scenario. We assumed all would go well, but what if it didn't? Heading into that day we were acutely aware of exactly how much trust we had put in another human being.

"Well, I don't think we have to worry about that. There's no reason not to feel good about this," Sara reassured us. In the past few months I had grown to know Sara in more than just the capacity of being our attorney. It was clear to me that besides representing us, she understood the years of heartache and disappointment we had endured.

I briefly researched the question myself and knew that

the number of cases where there was a legal problem between surrogacy parties was low. We had, after all, chosen the surrogacy route because we hoped it would alleviate any concern that the birth mother would change her mind. In fact, data from a 2002 review of approximately fifteen thousand surrogacy arrangements indicated an overall dispute rate of only .005 percent. Interestingly, that rate included even intended parents who had changed their minds, so in theory the number of cases involving conflict would seem even lower.[4]

Finally, in June of 2007, joined by our attorneys, Kevin, Ella, and I quietly and privately met in the Superior Court of Cobb County for the order of declaratory judgment.

The event went as smoothly as we all could have hoped, and it was again a special and momentous day for our family. For on that day, the baby boy growing inside of Ella's body legally became ours. Moving forward, should she go into labor at any point, we would have the right to make decisions with regard to the care of our baby, no questions asked.

Maybe I'm a mush, but I got teary-eyed in the proceedings, and trust me, I was doing everything I could to temper my emotions. To me, this legal hurdle wasn't something to be taken lightly. Every step was a piece of the puzzle that got us one milestone closer to the ultimate prize—a healthy newborn baby in our arms whom we could call our own.

As usual, Ella conducted herself with grace and poise during the proceeding, and I continued to be impressed with how she always allowed us to feel like this baby was ours. Her

---

4   What Happens If the Surrogate Changes Her Mind?;
http://www.surrogates-eggdonors.com/index.php?view=article&id=98

heart never wavered, and to this day I am grateful for not only the gift of carrying our child, but the generous, devoted, self-sacrificing, and loving spirit in which she delivered him to us.

NINETEEN

THINGS AREN'T ALWAYS
BLACK AND WHITE

The last couple of months of Ella's pregnancy were a little rocky. Dr. Miller didn't like the fact that the baby wasn't showing much growth, so he put Ella on a limited form of bed rest. The baby was measuring small, much as Tyler had toward the end of his gestation. As some concern for intrauterine growth restriction (IUGR) was growing, a date to induce labor was selected.

In the meantime, as the end of the pregnancy grew near, my sweet neighbors and friends threw us a baby shower. It was again a most unusual shower, since the mother-to-be was not actually pregnant. However, just as I had a few years before, I took great pleasure in the event, and was able to be more engaged in this shower, since I was not on bed rest for a change. I felt so lucky to have a considerate and loving group surrounding me, taking part in the celebration of our miracle in the making.

In the early morning of July 19, Ella checked into the hospital; she was joined by her fiancé, Anthony. Anthony was not yet a father, so he was about to get the experience of a lifetime. Kudos to him for loving Ella so much that he supported her through the surrogacy process and the birth of a child that, of course, wasn't even his. Without my knowing Anthony particularly well, he struck me as a sweet and calm-natured man, and he always greeted us with a warm smile. His presence was an obvious help to Ella, and we were glad he was there to assist her on this epic day. Tyler was at our house with his grandparents. They were all eagerly awaiting the news of a little brother.

The hospital staff had clearly been informed that we were the legally intended parents, so Kevin and I received hospital identification bracelets upon check-in. The room was busy with anticipation from the four of us, all wondering when things would begin to happen. At first the oxytocin was slow to kick in. Kevin and I were asked to leave the room as Dr. Cohen checked to see how much Ella was dilated. He eventually decided to turn up the drugs a notch, and sure enough, the contractions intensified, coming on steadily. Dr. Cohen excused us one more time as he checked Ella. We were quickly called back into the room, and she was ready to push the baby out. Anthony, Kevin, and I surrounded Ella and tried as best as we could to do what we were told.

For the remainder of her labor, Kevin and Anthony stood at the head of the bed together.

Kevin looked at Anthony, and in an effort to break the tension in the room, he joked, "If this baby comes out looking like you we're going to have a real problem!" We assumed Ella had been required to abstain from intercourse during at least parts of the fertility process, and we were moments away from determining whether she had indeed complied.

It provoked a chuckle from everyone, and then we got back to business. Ella was a pro, and due to the fact that she'd delivered two other children, combined with our baby's small size, things moved along rapidly.

In three short, seemingly easy pushes, our son arrived into this world. Our precious baby boy was finally here! Ella had done it for us—delivered the most wonderful and miraculous gift of all: the gift of life. I instantly thought to myself, *How will I ever truly be able to repay Ella for what she has done? There are no words of gratitude meaningful enough to express our thanks.*

In the meantime, the nursing staff was busy making sure the baby was doing well. His due date was originally in August, so his early arrival in July had everybody scrambling to make sure his stats were on track. The nurse at the warming table was performing her normal routine—weighing, cleaning, and evaluating the baby—when she paused for a moment and seemed somewhat disoriented.

I quickly asked, "Is something wrong?"

The nurse replied as she shook herself out of her momentary confusion, "Everything's fine. I'm just not used to Mom standing here as well."

To our great relief, the baby's health looked good.

Only a minute later, one of the other nurses quietly came over to me and put her hands on my shoulders.

She said to me in a low whisper, "You must tell me… *exactly* how did this happen?"

If the nurse had just thought about it for a moment, she could have understood what had happened medically. But in that moment she thought her eyes were fooling her.

I explained, "We are the biological parents, and Ella has given us the gift of being our gestational surrogate."

You could see the wires reconnecting in her brain as that made complete sense to her, and she mumbled something along the lines of "Ah, yes!" as she walked away and got back to work.

Admittedly it was a bit odd, seeing a stark white baby boy emerge from a black woman's body. There were only a handful of us in the room who expected it. Although Ella, Anthony, Kevin, and I had never talked about the difference in our races, it was, even for us, a truly incredible experience to witness this miracle of both science and faith!

The four of us marveled at our little guy for quite some time. We all took turns holding him and loving on him. Ella looked fabulous for having just given birth, and I was finally at ease that it had been a quick delivery and all appeared to have gone well for her. She looked comfortable and indicated that she felt well. She had received an epidural earlier in the day to help with the pain of the contractions. A look of satisfaction filled Ella's face. She had completed her goal for herself and for us; there was no mistaking the sense of relief that enveloped the room.

We discussed his name and told her we'd decided on Andrew Scott Urrutia; we planned to call him Drew. In the weeks leading up to his birth, we had been torn between Andrew and Austin. Ella preferred Andrew, and after her carrying him for us, it was important that she weigh in on the discussion. And so, rather than Artie Fisty, as Tyler had suggested only a few months before, we gave our newly arrived son a more traditional name.

Some parents pray their children will fulfill all their hopes and dreams after they are born. Our children had fulfilled ours just by being born. We now had two little earth angels who had arrived into this world safe and sound. The years to come would feel like a bonus.

TWENTY

MEET 50G

It's hard for me to describe the first few hours of life with Drew. My brain almost blocked out the minute details of the events due to how emotionally overwhelmed I felt by the experience of it all. I was thankful for his safe arrival, eternally grateful to Ella, and wrapped up in taking care of a newborn—and we had *lots* of visitors for this second miracle child! The staff at Northside Hospital were once again amazing to us. They made it clear that if they had a room, they would allow me to stay on the floor along with other new mothers. That way I could be with Drew through the night and take care of him, as if I had delivered him.

We were fortunate that they did have the space, and I was able to spend the night in a room only a few doors down from Ella. That was particularly nice, because it meant I could easily share Drew with her. I made regular visits to check on how she was feeling, and it gave both Ella and Anthony some time to snuggle with Drew. He was a tiny baby, weighing in at only five pounds (just as Tyler had). Drew looked healthy and strong despite his petite size. As an experienced mother, Ella was clearly comfortable holding him, but I was impressed with how at ease Anthony was with taking him as well.

Those first few days were filled with several unknowns for us. First and foremost on my mind, I wasn't sure how the transition would be for Ella. Having been Drew's carrier for the past nine months, she might find it extremely difficult to simply hand the baby over to us as planned. And understandably so. While it was all arranged in an agreed-upon manner, and with the legal backing to support it, it's just something one cannot take for granted. But as I have said before, Ella expressed nothing but the most sincere and heartfelt desire to give us this beautiful child in the most gracious manner. Both the accomplishment of carrying Drew and the way she comported herself throughout the process were tremendous gifts. It's funny, but having not been able to bear children well myself, one of the things I wish I could do for others is give the gift of a child. It's the ultimate blessing. The act of carrying a baby for someone who cannot do so is without a doubt one of the most selfless, benevolent, and extraordinary things one human being can do for another.

The second-biggest topic on my mind was the issue of breast milk. Ella and I had discussed this ahead of time, and it was decided that we would give Drew formula. As mentioned earlier, this had not been an easy decision for me. Although I couldn't easily produce milk, I could have asked Ella to use a pump and collect breast milk. Eventually I concluded that I did not want her doing that for two reasons: One, it could possibly prolong any emotional attachment she might have to the baby, only making her separation harder. Two, it would certainly prolong her physical recovery. Having experienced the engorgement I had after the loss of Tess, I thought it was best that she not supply any breast milk and just be done with the pain of that in a few days. Plus, it would make her return to work and to her family much easier.

The last unknown for us was how Tyler would take to the idea of a little brother, especially after not having a pregnant mother. We assumed he would welcome his brother amicably, as most siblings would. We had included Tyler in many doctors' appointments, he had seen all the ultrasounds, and we talked about the baby constantly, making it a point to let him know he would soon be a big brother.

Tyler got to know Ella and her children fairly well, and I hoped that would also help him be comfortable with the surrogacy process. I figured he would one day play an important role in talking to his little brother about Ella and all that she did for us. I was pleased that not once did Tyler ask about the racial differences between Ella and us. It never occurred to him to "see" people by the color of their skin.

The moment Tyler laid eyes on Drew, he wanted to hold him and play with him. Adoringly, he called his baby brother "Lovey," and for quite a while that was the name Tyler preferred to use. We were all like one big, happy family in the hospital—our family of four, plus Ella and Anthony, then my parents, and also Kevin's parents came to visit. It was a celebration for our very long-awaited baby. And no one was about to miss out on that.

In one day, Ella was well enough to be released from the hospital; there was no need for her to stay, as most postpartum mothers would. She did not have a baby to take care of, so they discharged her faster than what would be typical. I gave her multiple hugs and I pray we adequately expressed the thanks she deserved. We made plans to be in touch soon, and to see each other in the upcoming weeks. I remained in the hospital until Drew was released. Interestingly, a few strange looks had already come my way—looks that implied confusion at the fact that I was caring for a newborn but clearly didn't look like I had just carried a baby on my five-foot-two, hundred-pound frame for the past nine months.

During one of my first adventures out of the house after Drew's birth, I had an interaction with a total stranger that I will never forget. I was walking through a local mall, headed to the indoor playground with the boys. Tyler was so excited to be going. He was used to more playtime than he had gotten in the past week. Drew was only about seven days old. As we approached the indoor play area, we paused to get a bottle ready for Drew so I could feed him while Tyler played. A woman came over to me. I expected her to look at our new baby and ask about him, as strangers often take delight in admiring newborns.

To my amazement, she glared at me with a bit of an attitude. "How old is your baby?" she asked.

"He's just a week old," I said with a proud smile, looking down at the miracle in my arms.

She immediately began to insult me. "You bitch!" she exclaimed. "I can't believe you just had a baby a few days ago and you look like that." She couldn't contain the words in her mouth as she stared me up and down.

I refused to let that one sit. On behalf of adoptive and "intended" mothers everywhere who would have given their left arm to carry a baby to term, I started my rebuttal.

"Did it ever occur to you that parents might acquire babies in a variety of ways? Some give birth, some adopt, and some have surrogate mothers when they are not able to get pregnant or carry a baby themselves. Could you for a moment have stopped and thought about the fact that I certainly don't look like I carried this baby? If you just considered that there might be another option, you never would have said something so rude to me. I would have happily gained a permanent twenty pounds carrying my child. You have absolutely no idea how much we went through to have this baby."

She was clearly taken aback. "I'm s-s-sorry," she stammered.

You should be, lady. I finished making the bottle for Drew and escorted Tyler into the playground. It occurred to me then that I had received some similar unkind looks from women in the hospital, or confused looks from their husbands, as they tried to decipher the combination of my petite, thin frame in conflict with the newborn in my arms. It was such an ironic consequence. I had felt (admittedly I'm not proud of my emotions) jealous of all the women who could carry a baby full-term, and here was a woman jealous of me simply because I didn't have some leftover baby weight to shed? If she only understood what we had gone through to arrive at this place.

My first few months home with Drew were, to be completely candid, really rough. While I could not have been happier to have another baby in our home, he was an infant who had terrible reflux. Truly awful reflux. I was changing his clothes sometimes five and six times a night because he was spitting up so much. His pain level with the reflux was intense throughout his infancy, and he would cringe with his knees pulled to his chest. The discomfort would last for hours while he cried most of the night. We saw a gastroenterologist and tried multiple medicines, but nothing really seemed to relieve the pain. He was somewhat better during the daytime, and especially when he was held upright, so we contrived a couple alternative sleeping options for the first four months of his life. We began with putting his infant-to-toddler rocker in his crib, and resting him in that. It had a foot piece that allowed it to be stabilized. As he got older and shifted around more, we put a wedge under the crib mattress to elevate his upper body.

When Drew was a newborn, Kevin took a job at another medical device company. He was on the road almost nonstop with a position as a sales manager for the state of Florida. His travel schedule intensified due to several months of training with his new employer. This was followed by a solid year of recruiting to ramp up his new team. His trips regularly took him all over the United States rather than keeping him local to the Southeast. While he missed seeing the boys, I wondered whether he welcomed sleeping in a hotel most nights during this phase of our lives—Kevin did not deal well with repeated disruptions in his sleep. I felt something like a single parent, especially Monday through Friday. I was at the height of my sleep deprivation, and you could have easily referred to me as a walking zombie. Drew's feeding schedule as a lightweight combined with his reflux had me getting fifteen-minute catnaps even through the night. Tyler kept me busy all day long, since he was such an active little toddler. He had given up his naps by the time he was two years old. I was eager for Tyler's Mother's Morning Out program to begin. Having him at "school" meant that I would get a few hours' relief and perhaps squeeze in a nap while Drew slept.

My friend Allison once again came to my rescue. She told me to hang in there and that Drew should begin to get better at the ten-week mark. Things seemed to improve a little then, but even a little felt like a lot. He made further strides again at four months. At that point we slept Drew flat in the crib and went into hard-core sleep-training mode. When his reflux wasn't bothering him, he was an absolute joy.

Once the reflux subsided, you could decipher his true personality, which was that of a child who was just happy to be here. Under any circumstances, Drew wanted to be a part of the action. He was easygoing and funny from a very early age. For as small as he was initially, he quickly began to make up for it. When Drew was about six months old, the symptoms of his reflux greatly subsided when he was allowed to eat table food. He started gaining weight, growing, and eating like a champ. He had a tremendous appetite, and loved everything I put on his plate. He ate huge portions of healthy foods. I soon learned I could give him the meals Kevin and I ate simply by chopping or mashing our foods very finely.

On one of Kevin's first adventures out of the house with Drew, he had a memorable conversation as well. He took Drew with him to do a little grocery shopping. As he was walking through the store, he bumped into a neighbor. She peered excitedly at Drew while he slept in his car seat.

"Oh, wow! I see you guys finally had the baby! He's so cute. What's his name?"

I'm not sure what came over Kevin, but true to his sense of humor he replied, "Well, have you heard of the rapper 50 Cent?"

She paused, gave him a confused look, and said, "Yes…"

"Well, meet my son 50G."

She laughed, but with a little uncertainty.

He clarified, "Our surrogacy experience was kind of expensive."

Then it clicked for her that Kevin was referring to the approximate amount of money we had spent to get Drew here.

I knew that in reality we both considered him priceless. He was worth much more than the "50G" nickname he had earned. But it was a funny name nonetheless, and it helped put us at ease about the financial undertaking it had been to bring this child into our lives.

From the very beginning Drew has adored his big brother, and the two of them have a beautiful and typically sometimes feisty sibling relationship. With that said, their love for each other is obvious, and they are keenly aware of the missing sister in their lives. Kevin, Tyler, and I occasionally talk about Tess, and as Drew grows older, he learns more about her and the circumstances leading to her loss. We have always been honest with Drew that I did not carry him in my body. It's a discussion that is repeated every once in a while, as needed, for clarification. The older he gets, the more details he wants both about how I lost Tess and how he was created. At first the conversations were simple.

"Mommy's body was not good at carrying babies anymore after losing baby Tess," I would explain. Candidly I reminded him, "You are here today because of the generosity of Ella, and what she did for us so that we could have you as our son!"

As he grew older the discussion included additional descriptions. "Drew, normally when a woman is pregnant, it takes about forty weeks for a baby to fully grow and develop inside his/her mommy's body. The baby is in a sac filled with a fluid, and this helps to keep the baby safe. At only twenty-two weeks into my pregnancy with Tess, my water broke, which means I got a tear in the sac and too much fluid leaked out to keep Tess alive in my body. I had to deliver her so much earlier than usual that she wasn't able to survive. It was nature's way of telling me that it wasn't okay for me to carry babies anymore, which is what led us to look for another woman whose body was capable of safely carrying a baby for us."

Each time, he is increasingly mesmerized by the story, and his awareness for the miracle of life grows with it. Many people who meet Drew tell me he has an old soul, and I believe his appreciation for how he arrived into this world has deeply affected his character.

When Drew was only a baby, I took him to see Ella every few months. Around the time he was a year old, life began to get busier for both of us. The in-person visits became stretched farther apart, and eventually Ella moved to another state and we relocated from Alpharetta to Greensboro, Georgia. We remain in touch, and I send pictures of Drew to her so she can see the great rewards of her hard work, dedication, and act of selflessness.

You would think that since Tyler is such a prolific talker it might stifle Drew's ability to speak up in our household. Luckily he has held his own and, much like Tyler, he was unusually verbal very early on. He has grown up to be a little social charmer among his classmates (or so I am told by his teachers).

Most important, it is evident to me that his greatest gift is something we have never had to teach him. It is his inherent kindness and generosity to others...much like the woman who carried him.

REMEMBERING TESS

January 12, 2012

Dear family and friends:

I am writing this on what would be Tess's sixth birthday. I am inspired to share a few thoughts with you.

The sadness and grief I feel today are as acute and fresh as the day she died. Those words, "sadness" and "grief," are merely shallow descriptions. The aching inside me is far more gut-wrenching than that. There are no appropriate words.

This coming Saturday we will baptize Drew. Planning for it made me reflect on the other two children we have baptized. Tyler's service was traditional in every way. For Tess, the priest in the hospital asked whether he could use the tears rolling down our cheeks as the water to baptize her. He collected them in a small seashell, which I still have today.

This year I plan to share with Tyler the handprints and footprints we have of Tess, maybe a few photos, and other precious keepsakes. He has asked for years to see them, and I think it's finally time. Or maybe I am just finally ready. I think I have waited to show him, ironically, because he seems to comprehend it so well. It is a hard reality that people don't always die in the natural order of things. And yet he already understands that the "natural order" is really God's order, the way in which His divine plan unfolds. It does not necessarily match what we are taught or what we expect.

And so, on this day, perhaps take a few extra moments to hug your child/children and tell them again just how very much you love them. Don't rush it. Oddly, it is hard for me to remember exactly how many hours Tess lived on the day she was born. But in the short time she was alive and even after she passed, we held her for the rest of that day and into the night, telling her over and over that we loved her. I stared through my tears at her small, perfect body, her hand gripping my finger. Even then, she resembled Tyler. I cradled her and caressed her, aching for her to know I was her mother in the short time we had together, desperate for her to know how much we loved her.

My belief in heaven has grown stronger since Tess's passing. Whether real or manufactured, it is a way for me to know I will see her again, hold her again, be with her again, tell her I love her again. The time we had together was simply not enough. There are so many would-haves, could-haves, should-haves...and yet there will never be any of them with her on earth.

In Tess's birth/death announcement, we reminded people to count their blessings, and I do that here today. Each of you is a blessing to me, and I am grateful for all that I receive from you. You help to give me strength, especially on days like this.

Love and hugs,
Stacey

TWENTY-ONE

SEEING THE GIFTS THROUGH
THE SCARS THAT REMAIN

So, how does all of this impact our lives now? The pressure to bring a child into this world is a thing of the past. Both of our boys are now school age, and our concerns in having them have been replaced with different worries—ones that are typical for anyone raising children. The journey to make our family, however, has left its mark in many different ways.

First of all, we have learned through experience that families are created in more than one traditional way—through IVF, adoption, surrogacy, foster parenting, etc. Those children are all loved the same. In fact, I would venture to say that sometimes families who "work harder" for their children might feel as though they appreciate them more. Certainly those who have easy pregnancies would not agree; without argument their children are loved equally as much. But, for many of us who struggle to have a family, the journey we take has been a consuming portion of our adult lives. Even after the struggle ends, the memory of it remains with us. Every morning when my children awake, I see the gift of their presence. The losses of my past make me acutely aware that I need to live in the moment. I am all too cognizant that their lives could end prematurely, and while I don't anticipate that, I am conscious of it.

Kevin and I are both extremely vocal in our love for our children. We never hesitate to show our affection with hugs, kisses, and snuggles, regardless of their ages. I have no doubt that our boys know how intensely they are loved and how hard we worked to have them. They are aware of the challenges we faced, and by sharing our story honestly with them we've helped them become sensitive to our past and to other people who may be struggling to start a family. I think the health-care providers who helped us bring our children safely into this world also appreciate our journey. While they may not personally experience the pain, I do believe that thoughtful physicians, nurses, and technicians become a part of the journey with each family. After Drew was born, we received a beautiful little hand-painted chair from Dr. Miller, the perinatologist who worked with us during most of my pregnancies. I thought it was particularly kind of him and his wife, considering the hundreds, if not thousands of patients he sees. It's a gift we have cherished, not only because it represents the birth of Drew, but it reminds us of the compassion from the health-care professionals who also took part in our story.

There are plenty of ways our journey has had an effect

on our everyday lives. For instance, when Tyler was younger, he would draw family pictures. In his simple stick-figure sketches there would be five of us, because he always included Tess.

I mentioned that Tyler was a chatty and talkative young fellow. Well, as a toddler, when I pushed him around in a grocery cart, he would very easily engage people in conversation. Frequently he would tell strangers in the store that he had a little sister but she died. Yes, it was awkward, but mostly for the stranger. We were used to talking about her.

He would tell kids and teachers at school that he had a sister, but then they would never see her, so I learned at the beginning of the school year to explain the situation to the teacher. That way, in case he spoke of her (or her passing), or drew pictures of her, they were prepared to handle it with him or with the other children in class. Likewise, when Drew is asked whether he has any brothers or sisters, he will occasionally inform new friends that he has a brother and he had a sister, but she died. I am always eager to jump in and explain her loss in simple terms. I can see the confused look on children's faces when they learn a baby has died. It's a lot for a child to comprehend, and especially without the comfort of their parents to put them at ease with such inconceivable news.

Now that Tyler is older, he always remembers her birthday, to the point that he preps me for it.

"Mom, this is Tess's birthday week," he says in a voice that is soft and sweet, but proud that he is reminding me. Little does he know…How could I ever forget? But it warms my heart that he needs no reminder. He realizes now that it is not generally socially acceptable to discuss her, because of the discomfort it brings to others. He has learned to be more tactful about how and when he brings up the subject. Drew is still learning how to handle the topic.

❦

On a beautiful fall afternoon, when Tyler was only a kindergartner, Kevin and Tyler went on a long walk. Kevin was in a particularly pensive mood. They talked about a variety of things, and just enjoyed spending some time outside together. Kevin could sense that Tyler was also a little heavyhearted. As the two of them drew near our home, Tyler finally admitted what had been weighing on his mind.

"Daddy, I really miss Tess." And then, with a reassurance and maturity at only five years old that we admired, he continued. "But it's okay. She'll always be in my heart."

"Mine too, buddy. Mine too," Kevin responded.

Maybe it's because Tyler is a firstborn child, or it's just in his nature, or it's because we had a lot of sobering issues going on when he was young, but he is our more serious child. He can be hilarious at times, but his approach to life is more deliberate. He is a fiercely competitive child, bound and determined to succeed in all aspects of his day. From school to sports to a game of cards, there is no letting down his guard. Knowing that about him now has always made me wonder whether that tenacity is what helped him make it through the womb despite his horrendous odds.

On the other hand, he is a completely sensitive child

too, never giving up the opportunity to snuggle with us one more time before bed, or again first thing in the morning. He cares what his friends say to him, and what they think of him. He's not a boy who lets things slide easily off his shoulders. He tells Kevin and me every day how much he loves us; in fact, both boys do…and it's the most wonderful gift we could ever receive. They regularly say, "You're the best mom/dad ever!" and battle with us over who loves whom more.

I pray that doesn't ever end. I know one day I won't be so popular in their eyes. Tyler is a sweet child who tells me I'm pretty and stops to fix my hair or notice that I've made the bed with different linens. I believe he is already conscientious of how special he is to us. As he gets older, he has begun to understand some of the physical and logistical aspects of what we went through to have him, and he further appreciates our love for him.

I had a rare gift this past Valentine's Day. As we were ready to walk out the door for school in the morning, I turned and paused, squatted down low, and peered into Tyler's eyes.

With a slight smile on my face, I said in a prodding voice, "Who is your Valentine today? Is there anyone special you have in mind?"

He had informed me earlier that some of the boys in his class were giving individual Valentine cards or gifts to girls they had crushes on. I was curious whether he secretly liked someone.

"You are my Valentine, Mom. I love you the most," he said. I just about melted on the spot.

"I love you, too, buddy. That makes me the happiest mom in the whole world to hear you say that. You know I'm the luckiest mom around, don't you?"

And we began our game: "Well, I'm the luckiest kid to have you and Dad...."

"Okay, get your backpack and head to the car."

It was my turn with Drew now. I stopped him as he wrapped up brushing his teeth and we exchanged a Valentine hug.

"Do you have a special Valentine today, Drew? Is there any one person you'd like to have for your Valentine?"

"Well, it's you, Mom. You are my Valentine!" He looked at me as if it were silly that I should ask. He rolled his eyes at me and flashed the cute smile that could only be his. I told him how much he meant to me as well.

I was two for two. With tears in my eyes, I explained to Kevin later that it just doesn't get any better than that. How many years will I be so lucky? How many years will my boys pick me as their Valentine? For most of their youth they are either too young to care or they will get old enough to have a crush on a girl in their class. Then they will be dating someone, then they will be engaged, and then they will be married. And Mom is never again their Valentine.

It's not to be taken lightly. I was on top of the world. My angels made my day and more.

This is the stuff my dreams are made of.

~

Every night, as I put the boys to bed, I ask them about the best and worst part of their day. We call it our "peak" and our "pit"; it was an idea we inherited from some of our dear friends who live in Tennessee. It's a nice way to revisit the goings-on of the day and address any issues the kids have on their minds before bedtime.

This night was no different. We had spent the afternoon in the tiny nearby town of Bostwick, Georgia. Tyler played in a scrimmage baseball game, and the kids were exhausted, so I got straight to the point as I tucked Drew in first.

"Okay, Drew," I began. "Let's hear it. Give me your peak and your pit."

"Well, I can tell you my pit right away. Did you know there was a baby in one of those graves today? He lived for only three days," he said with compassion.

The baseball field had been directly next to the town cemetery, and the younger siblings of all the players weaved their way through the cemetery as the game was being played. From the bleachers I had noticed Drew in the graveyard, still as a statue, peering down at a particular headstone. His hands rested on his hips and his head was cocked to the side. Finally some of the other children joined him. Although Drew was only five, he could read what it said, and one of the older children calculated the age of the child whose name appeared on the headstone.

"Yes, I know. I saw that, too. His name was Little Joe." It had been hard to miss. Among all the larger, prominent headstones stood a petite one, and it almost screamed out to me. I had immediately thought of Tess, and my heart ached for the parents who had lost a child as well.

"You know what is a nice thought about Little Joe, Drew? I bet your sister, Tess, is playing with him up in heaven. So as much as his parents miss him here on earth, we know he has a great playmate where he is now, right?"

"He sure does," Drew said with some relief.

"How about if we say a prayer now for Tess and Little Joe? And we can ask God to make sure he's taking good care of both of them for us. We can also ask God to watch over his parents and make sure they're doing okay. It must be hard for parents to lose a child after only three days, don't you think?"

Drew nodded his head up and down with sincerity. So we said our prayers together that night, and Drew seemed at peace.

My children have learned a life lesson that I did not fully realize and appreciate until much, much later: The sequence in which we die does not always occur in the manner we are taught it should happen.

Both of our children are sensitive and conscientious of life and of others. They know death can come at any time. Allison and Steve Carr's children do too. They remember Tess in the same way, and are aware that sometimes even babies die.

The Carrs' second child, Maggie, said, "If we hadn't lost Tess we might not have had the chance to know Drew."

Somehow it seems so innocent and kind when said from a child's perspective. Maggie is the daughter Allison was carrying when we lost Tess. When I look at her I can't help but think of Tess and how they would have been playmates. What Maggie accomplishes is my landmark for where Tess would have been.

And as for Drew, it's as though part of Tess lives within him. He is truly angelic. He has an innate sense of humor and a charming way with others. He is loving and considerate in the most generous of ways. Drew is the kind of kid who, when he gets handed a cookie and discovers he loves it, will save the remainder of it to share with those around him rather than enjoying it all himself.

If a friend is hurt, he is genuinely concerned. There isn't a lazy bone in his body; he even helps me cook and clean the house. If I get my hair done, he notices. When I get dressed up, he tells me I look beautiful. He adores animals and all things in nature. He is an avid lizard hunter and collector of creatures.

He is a true lover and protector of life. And I think there is no irony in that. He already knows he wants to be a doctor, and I believe there's a strong chance he will become one. His compassion for others is palpable. He is an authentic caregiver, which in my opinion is something that can't be taught. He's going to make some lady very happy one day.

Another amusing and pressure-filled result of our unusual baby-making story in this house has been the requirement to talk about "the birds and the bees" somewhat earlier than usual. Tyler, by the age of six, wanted to know how Drew was made, and by the age of nine he flat-out demanded that he know how he himself was created. He understood there were major differences, and realized that I carried him and another woman carried Drew. So, scientifically, there just had to be some explanation to satisfy his curiosity.

The four of us were gathered around the dinner table one night when Tyler laid it on the line.

"I want to know how a baby is made. Please tell me *now*."

For fear that the inquisition would continue in front of Drew, Kevin struck a deal then and there.

"We will agree to tell you, but not here at the dinner table. I promise we will talk about it within the next two weeks," he said, which satiated Tyler for the time being.

It was a conversation that took place soon after, fortunately in private and without five-year-old Drew, who was not yet ready for that detailed discussion.

By pure coincidence, not long after that, Drew and I had a somewhat similar conversation that morphed into a much more meaningful exchange, one I will never forget.

Somehow our nightly peak-and-pit talk slowly turned to the topic of Tess and subsequently to having babies. He asked me to remind him about the various ways babies can be born. He recalled that Tyler was "cut out of my belly" via a C-section, and then, at the advice of a close friend, I refreshed his memory of a talk we had once before.

"Remember, Drew, that women have three holes down

in their private area: one for going pee-pee, one for going poo-poo, and one for delivering babies." *Keep it simple. The basics are all he needs.* I was giving him more information than many other parents would, but I believed in answering the question and being honest.

"Well, how did you make me, though? I mean, how did you get me from your body to Ella's?" he inquired. He deserved to know.

"That is a great question, buddy. It's a little complicated for me to answer, but I will try my best to explain it." I went on in the exact way we had attempted to explain it to Tyler years before.

Prior to giving my "How to Make a Baby via Surrogate 101" class, I gave Drew a caveat.

"The only reason I'm willing to share these details with you now is because I think you are old enough and mature enough to finally hear them." He had just celebrated his sixth birthday. In addition, I asked him for assurance that he would not disclose the information to *any* of his friends.

I reiterated, "Remember, this is something children discuss only with their parents." *At least, let's hope so for now.*

I began, "Mommy's body, as you know, was not good at carrying babies. So, what the doctor did was take an egg from my body and a cell from Daddy's body and put them together in a special dish, called a petri dish." I decided to use the word "cell" instead of "sperm." If he did tell any of this to a friend, it would at least be G-rated.

I continued. "Then, when the egg and cell join together, they begin to make a baby, and that baby was *you*. The developing baby is called an 'embryo,' and it starts to divide, first into two cells, then into four cells, and then into eight cells. When you were only eight cells big, they transferred you from the petri dish into Ella's body, so that she could carry you for me. She gave us the gift of you! Isn't that amazing?"

Drew's eyes grew bigger as he listened in complete astonishment. He was taking it all in and couldn't believe what he was hearing.

"Once you were in her body, your cells kept dividing and you kept growing until you were ready to live as a baby outside of her. We were with her when she gave birth to you in the hospital, and we brought you home with us."

"So she gave me the gift of life, didn't she?" he said. I instantly choked up, because I knew right away that he got it. In that very moment it totally clicked for him. He knew he was alive today because of the generosity and willingness of another woman to carry him for us.

"Yes, sweetie, that's right. Isn't that just the most awesome gift? Isn't it incredible that she would do that for us? Without Ella, we wouldn't have you."

And then he wore a look of panic.

"Mama"—he called me that sometimes—"what if Ella wasn't able to carry me? Would you have found someone else to carry me?"

And then it hit me like a ton of bricks: Drew was always supposed to exist. It wasn't just *any* embryo that was supposed to make it. It was specifically Drew, and he, of course, knew that. This little child of mine and child of God already had it figured out way ahead of me. In his mind it was perfectly clear:

There was no option for him not to exist. No world without him in it. He was always meant to be. Always a part of a divine plan. It was so plain and simple for him to see. I could not imagine our lives without Drew. Yet why did it take my hearing this from him before I could come full circle and acknowledge that the loss of Tess did indeed give us the love of Drew? Thinking of it in this light was a true revelation for me.

"Drew, Daddy and I never would have stopped searching until we found someone to carry you. We would have looked and looked and looked until we found just the right person to make sure we could have you. It's part of why you and your brother are so extra-special. For some people it's very easy to have children, and that is great and wonderful and they are very lucky. But you should know that you are so wanted and so loved. We prayed for a long time and worked extremely hard to have both of you."

"I'm glad about that," was his simple response. "I love you, Mommy."

"I love you too, Drew."

As I started to understand the bigger purpose behind our journey—knowing and accepting that all along God had a plan—I became more in tune with the spiritual road I was traveling. I was on a much-improved path to a relationship with God—the key word being "relationship." The more I acknowledge Christ in me and in my life, the more I realize how shallow my relationship with Him was before. The conversation with Drew was one that flipped a switch in my brain. It turned me on and lit me up in such a way that I began to better interpret the heartache of our story as a gift. It was a key moment in the transition from feeling anger and resentment toward a God who I felt had betrayed me to a loving, omniscient God who was trying to teach me through this journey of pain, loss, and desperation.

Kevin and I were raised going to church. For both of us, particularly in our youth as our faith was being shaped, we had some very negative interactions within the churches we attended. For Kevin, there were church leaders who embezzled money and molested young children. For me, the experience included going to confession, only to be confronted later in front of a group of peers regarding the very things each of us had confessed. There was no element of trust for us within our churches. As a result, we struggled to feel spiritually satisfied. We stopped going to church for a long period of time. We eventually decided that rather than worrying about the label of the religion, and the guilt that was associated with a departure from the church we were raised in, it was far more important to find the growth and fulfilling spiritual guidance we were seeking. Our children began asking for more religious structure also, and that was all we needed to find a more appropriate solution for us and for our family.

In short, we began attending what I would describe as a nondenominational church. It has been a complete and radical change from what we were accustomed to, but I will make this one statement: In only a few short months, I learned more about the Bible and felt more inspired to have a better relationship with God than I had in the past forty years. It was incredibly rewarding to my husband and me. The bonus was that our children felt better about it too. They attended children's church during the services for adults. They learned about God on a level that was better adjusted to their age. Consequently, I stand firm in my belief that people should seek out a church that is the right fit for them, whatever that may be. I am confident that God does not care about the denominational label under which I pray to Him, and if anything, He would be happy with the progress I continue to make in my faith journey.

The other spiritual instruction I have really begun to appreciate over the past year is from the teachings of Pastor Andy Stanley, founder of North Point Ministries. He is the senior pastor at North Point Community Church (NPCC), located in Alpharetta, Georgia. We used to live about one mile from the church and, ironically, never attended. My next-door neighbor regularly invited us to services there, but Kevin and I were not ready to explore something different yet. After hearing about what a dynamic speaker he was, I ventured online to take a look for myself. His sermons are available in multiple formats. His online recordings were ideal for a person like me, living in Greensboro, Georgia, which was nearly two hours away from the NPCC campus. After listening to only a few series, I was hooked.

I find his style appealing because the message is so relatable. In fact, he often talks about how the NPCC goal is to create a church that unchurched people love to attend, and as a result his messages appeal to the masses. He provides practical commentary on how to lead a good and purposeful life. Even non-Christians can benefit from what he preaches, but he does enhance and support his sermons with biblical scriptures. I am better able to comprehend and absorb the words of the Bible when I learn about it with his assistance. Our family currently attends one of the NPCC satellite church programs available in our area.

The practice of a religion is, of course, a very personal thing. I will admit that during much of my infertility experiences I wasn't always able to lean on religious beliefs because I had so many doubts during the process. I relied on a strong will and stubborn tenacity to make it through our journey. For some people, digging deep and finding that inner strength is enough, and I can understand that. Our disappointments often fueled me to work even harder and become even more determined to figure out a way for us to bear children. But in the end, having children alone wasn't enough. For me, the spiritual component was a necessary ingredient to bring harmony into my life again.

Over time, through my own efforts and with the help of people like Andy, I began to have my own personal epiphany. When reflecting on my past, I realized that in my twenties and thirties I was totally focused on getting what I wanted out of my prayers to God. I was thinking selfishly. Now, by contrast, I am learning how to pray for living with Christ in me. As such, I recognize that the adversity bestowed upon me was a bigger part of God's plan. While it may have been very painful, I needed to learn that our journey was God's intention. I understand now that I could have, in the face of all of our struggles, made the choice to move farther away from God and my faith, or I could embrace the challenge and trust that He had a more important purpose for the pain.

And here's the benefit to this new way of thinking: I can apply this to all the obstacles in my life—past, present, and future. My toughest hardship so far may have been infertility related, but for other people, it may be their failing marriage, declining health, troubled finances…any number of things. With patience, hopefully, one can discover exactly what God's bigger plan was once one arrives on "the other side" of the painful time.

Most notably, until I learned to see our adversity as a gift, I was constantly struggling with it.

For example, after we had Tyler, and even after we had Drew, I remained somewhat despondent about losing Tess and our other babies. My ability to be happy was blurred by the black cloud of those events, and I became blind to the other joys and blessings in my life. For years, I lived with an undercurrent of anger in my life. Our story made me wonder how other people with perhaps even more difficult situations survived their journey. What about people who could never conceive, or didn't have the finances to pursue help through an infertility specialist or surrogacy and adoption? What about people who receive a cancer diagnosis and have no medical cure? How do they persevere through that and get to a place of peace prior to their death?

The answer for me has been to welcome adversity with open arms. This does not mean that I feel better because I have some sort of closure on the subject matter. There will never be closure to losing our babies. It is a loss that resides permanently in our hearts. Rather, I have learned to live with it more peacefully because I have discovered the value in my journey. First, it was crucial that I learned to accept what I didn't understand. Then I acknowledged that the path God put me on has a purpose and a promise of something greater. I recognized that my pain had a reward, the greatest of which was an extremely improved relationship with God. The other greater purpose behind my pain was the chance to share our story. By living through it, and surviving it, I can help others who may be on a similar journey. Being cognizant of the bigger picture makes our experience not only more palatable, but it actually teaches me to find thanksgiving in our odyssey.

Now that I am learning more about the Bible, I discovered that many of the people Jesus admired most experienced great suffering—suffering we can't even begin to comprehend in today's world. Who am I to think that I am better than that? Who am I to think that I should deserve a life free of hardship? If those whom Jesus loved the most maintained their faith despite their anguish, who am I to falter in my faith? Even Jesus himself did not avoid suffering. In fact, he experienced unthinkable pain for the sake of all of us. I certainly don't deserve to escape such pain. James, Jesus' brother, may have explained it best:

> "Consider it pure joy, my brothers and
> sisters, whenever you face trials of many kinds,
> because you know that the testing of your faith
> produces perseverance. Let perseverance finish its

work so that you may be mature and complete, not lacking anything."

James 1: 2-4 (NIV)

We will all have trials in our lives. Looking for something good in what initially seems miserable is the way up and out of the pain. I agonized for years to appreciate what good could come out of losing all those babies. How could I pull myself out of the grievous state I lived in? My family, and especially Tyler, and then Drew, gave me the hope to continue on. Faith endures trials, and the testing of my faith produced patience. If I had never been tested, I would never believe as strongly as I do today. And with that enduring faith, I should lack nothing. People who are mature in their faith have the ability to face adversity and rise above it. They learn to persevere against all odds. They believe in God despite their misfortunes, and come out on the other side of the battle with an even greater trust in Him. This is how we honor God the most, and in return, we receive the most from Him.

During the painful phase of any struggle, it may feel easier to quit. Once I realized God had another plan, I actually understood that gifts arise from the pain. Now my prayer for peace in my life has also led me to include a prayer for the wisdom to understand the past and to accept that God has His own plan in store for me. In a recent sermon from NPCC, the speaker made a point to emphasize that peace doesn't come with the resolution of the problems of the present (or the past, for that matter). It comes instead with the promise of His presence. I am learning to find trust in His presence alone.

I have made a concerted effort to openly talk about God in our home, and I hope I am having an impact on our children. Drew, in particular, is a really spiritual little fellow. He will be on an adventure walk through the woods, and stop to admire, as he says, "…all the beauty God created for us to enjoy." He is keenly aware of how awesome nature is, and has the ability to appreciate the fine details that many others take for granted, and he attributes this to God.

When I was putting him to bed one night, the depth of his understanding became obvious.

As I tucked him in, I said, "Good night, my perfect and precious little boy."

To which he replied, "Come on, Mom, you know I'm not perfect. Nobody is. The only one who's perfect is God."

In the back of my mind, I predicted he would give me that rebuttal, and I wanted him to understand my perspective.

"Well, you're right, Drew. God is the only one who is perfect. But *you* are perfect for *me*. I couldn't have asked for two more perfect children to be mine. It doesn't mean everything you do is perfect, but you and Tyler are everything I could have ever hoped and prayed for."

He seemed satisfied with my response, and in his usual adorable fashion, he said to me, "I love you equal." That was our current way of getting past the argument of who loved the other more.

I am content with the manner in which our children are learning about God. One of my biggest roles is to help them develop a level of trust in God that I lacked until I was in my forties. That way, as they face trials in their young lives, they can be better equipped to conquer that adversity. As for me, these days I am happy with the title of "believer." It seems a loving God would be pleased with that. In that role, I am now more able to love those around me, for all that He asks of me is to love others with the same compassion He has shown me. This, I think, is His ultimate wish for all of us.

It has taken me more than forty long years, but I have finally realized that I am not in control of my life. I can help steer it, but I am not the ultimate driver. That takes a lot for a person like me to admit. I've been getting there slowly but surely as I get older; perhaps I really am getting wiser. My six-year-old son made it so blatantly obvious that he was a part of God's plan—that he was always meant to exist. How could I ever doubt that, or question the timing of events as they unfold?

I should have known better than to try to negotiate with God in my early days, when I prayed diligently and specifically for a child. Is it possible that when I stopped being so definitive and tried praying more for peace, that is when He heard me best? I have also learned that part of embracing the fact that I am not in control means that I need to be thankful to God for both the good and the bad in my life. I may not always understand the path, but I need to trust that there is a reason for what transpires. I need to give in to that plan rather than resist it or fight it, as I have done previously.

As I listened to the sermon at church one Sunday, the message revealed how "God is never late." I reflected on my own story of what it took for us to have a family. I thanked God for the plan He had for us, the life He gave us. It was, after all, the perfect path.

TWENTY-TWO

THE BEAUTY IN MY FLAWS

Years ago, after our children were born, my grandmother sent me an e-mail one day with an interesting attachment. I'm not sure who the author of this inspirational Chinese proverb is, but it goes something like this:

There is an old story of an elderly Chinese woman who had two large pots. Each hung on the end of a pole, which she carried across her neck. One of the pots had a crack in it, while the other pot was perfect and always delivered a full portion of water.

At the end of the long walks from the stream to the house, the cracked pot arrived only half-full. For two years this went on daily, with the woman bringing home only one and a half pots of water.

Of course, the perfect pot was proud of its accomplishments. But the poor cracked pot was ashamed of its own imperfection, and miserable that it could do only half of what it had been made to do.

After two years of what it perceived to be bitter failure, it spoke to the woman one day by the stream.

"I am ashamed of myself, because this crack in my side causes water to leak out all the way back to your house."

The old woman smiled. "Did you notice that there are flowers on your side of the path, but not on the other pot's side? That's because I have always known about your flaw, so I planted flower seeds on your side of the path, and every day while we walk back, you water them. For two years now I have been able to pick these beautiful flowers to decorate the table. Without your being just the way you are, there would not be this beauty to grace the house."

The moral? Each of us has our own flaw. But it's the cracks and flaws that make individuals so unique, and make our lives together complementary. We've got to take each person for who he or she is and look for the good in them.

As a woman who has lost many pregnancies, I have an additional interpretation. This story really resonates with me. For a long time I had a hard time explaining to people why Drew is not a replacement for Tess.

Shortly after Drew was born, people would say, "If you hadn't lost Tess, you would never have Drew."

Or, "Now you have the two kids you were hoping for," this said as if Drew magically replaced Tess. My private response was, *Well, maybe. But that doesn't make it any easier on me. He doesn't replace her. He doesn't erase the pain of losing her. When you have a second child, do you forget about the first one you had? It doesn't work that way!*

But, of course, I would never say that out loud. Instead I would calmly explain that having Drew adds to our family as any new sibling would, but it doesn't mean we forget about Tess.

I loved this story about the old Chinese lady, because I am like the cracked pot, flawed in many ways, including the fact that I am essentially incapable of carrying babies. Out of my flaws we lost Tess, but traveled on our journey to have Drew...this beautiful, adorable, and amazing child who has been such a gift to us every day. We can't imagine our lives without Drew. He and Tyler "decorate" our lives in countless ways.

Out of a bad situation arose the good. Every person has a story and a struggle. After the loss of Tess, the birth of Drew was the encouragement I needed to continue to grow in my faith rather than deny it. I almost turned my back on my Creator, and that would have been a devastating path. I believe I would have continued a lifetime of underlying sadness and grief that blurred my vision for all the other blessings bestowed upon me.

It has been a long and difficult journey to feel as though our family is complete, but today indeed it is. We remember Tess each and every day. She is sometimes remembered with a smile and sometimes with tears. But at least in our home she is not forgotten. I pray that I will make it to heaven, where I will get to meet her, the rest of our angels, and others who have passed. For I long to tell Tess how sorry I am that my body failed her. I long for Tyler and Drew to eventually know their sister. And most of all, I long to hold her and tell her how dearly I love her, the way I have had the chance to tell my boys so many times.

Of course, by then, all will be forgiven. In heaven, the cracks in me will no longer matter.

It should be a very happy reunion.

ACKNOWLEDGMENTS

There are numerous people who deserve thanks for their supportive role in our lives as we endured the process of trying to make our family complete. For the sake of privacy, many shall remain anonymous, but hopefully they know who they are. A number of them were kind enough to read early versions of this book and then provide feedback to me in the most loving manner. A special thanks, in particular, goes to Dr. Lloyd B. Greig for his medical review and commentary. There are also countless doctors, nurses, technicians, and hospital/office staff who traveled this road with us and held our hands along the way. They were invaluable to our family. We recognize and appreciate that we were fortunate to have such an amazing array of health-care professionals—both private physician groups and the team at Northside Hospital—helping us through the medical aspect of our journey. The emotional support offered to us by the Northside Hospital Perinatal Palliative Care Program (specifically the H.E.A.R.T.strings Perinatal Bereavement Office) deserves equal praise, as they have continued to show compassion for our situation, even years after we lost Tess. For a tremendous amount of information as well as a comprehensive list of resources, I suggest visiting their site at http://www.northsidepnl.com. They offer free services to anyone, regardless of whether or not you were a patient at Northside Hospital.

I want to acknowledge Sara M. Clay, P.C., who acted as

our surrogacy attorney and provided a road map for us throughout the surrogacy process. Her passion and advocacy for helping prospective parents is indisputable.

Additionally, I offer my most sincere and heartfelt gratitude to my closest friends and family, especially to my parents and to Kevin's parents for the hours of care they gave me to ensure the safe delivery of their future grandchildren.

As a biology major and cancer researcher turned memoirist, I would like to thank both Tiffany Yates Martin of FoxPrint Editorial and Elise Daly Parker for their editorial reviews. Their expertise was crucial to educating me on how to be a better storyteller.

Finally, I would like to thank my husband, Kevin, for pushing me to write this book. As resistant as he once was to our more than difficult baby-making journey, there is now no one more grateful than he is for the two precious angels who grace our lives. His passion to have me share our story with others is derived from the insatiable appetite he has for spending time with our children. He, too, traveled on a spiritual journey that I believe could be learned only from our God-given experiences.